# Becoming an Effective Family Therapist

This book explores the link between the effectiveness of the family therapist and the complexity of the therapeutic relationship.

For family therapists the therapeutic alliance is complex because there are different family members, and the therapist must have an empathic relationship with each of them. Furthermore, the therapist is focused on facilitating the development of trust between the family members. The book highlights the family therapist not as an interventionist but as someone who is focused on establishing a good relationship with different family members. It includes research and theory as well as case studies, exploring topics such as: the therapist's emotion regulation, the therapist's inner dialogue, and dealing with client feedback. The main idea is simple but important: the goal of family therapy is not healing, but connection. A family therapist knows that connection heals. Connection also protects against suffering in the future.

This book is essential for beginning and seasoned family therapists, systemic therapists, and graduate students.

**Peter Rober** is a clinical psychologist and family therapist. He is professor at the Institute for Family and Sexuality Studies, Medical School (University of Leuven, Belgium). His research focus is on the psychotherapy process in family therapy, and on processes in families (trauma, grief, secrecy, etc.). He has numerous publications on these subjects in international peer-reviewed journals.

"What is this process of becoming a family therapist? How do we understand it? Peter Rober offers us a profound, thoughtful and compassionate exploration and description of how we become an effective family therapist for today's families and communities. Drawing on the available research and many examples from his long years of practice experience, Peter's wisdom and love of his work shines through every page of this practical textbook."

**Arlene Vetere,** *VID Specialized University, Oslo, Norway*

"In this superb book, Peter Rober helps the reader understand the essence of effective family therapy. Assiduously drawing from a variety of different traditions in family therapy, Rober immerses us in the experiential world of being and becoming a family therapist. The wisdom he transmits emphasizes learning specific methods and drawing from research, but also the book accentuates development of the self of the therapist to be able to be fully present in sessions. Filled with instructive and moving clinical vignettes, and with many easily applied methods, this is the best book I know for today's beginning family therapist and a must read for everyone else."

**Jay L. Lebow,** *Ph.D., ABPP, Senior Scholar and Clinical Professor, Family Institute at Northwestern and Northwestern University*

"An efficient and passionate book, written from the front lines of psychotherapy. Necessary book for everyone who is learning to do family therapy; essential book for those who really want to BE a family therapist."

**Valentín Escudero,** *Research Center for Systemic Interventions, University of A Coruña, Spain; director of the Family Therapy Program for Children and Adolescents at Risk*

# Becoming an Effective Family Therapist

## Research, Practice, and Case Stories

Peter Rober

Routledge
Taylor & Francis Group

LONDON AND NEW YORK

Designed cover image: imaginima © Getty Images

First published in English 2024
by Routledge
4 Park Square, Milton Park, Abingdon, Oxon OX14 4RN

and by Routledge
605 Third Avenue, New York, NY 10158

*Routledge is an imprint of the Taylor & Francis Group, an informa business*

© 2024 Peter Rober

First published in Dutch by Pelckmans 2023

*British Library Cataloguing-in-Publication Data*
A catalogue record for this book is available from the British Library

*Library of Congress Cataloging-in-Publication Data*
Names: Rober, Peter, author.
Title: Becoming an effective family therapist : research, practice and case stories / Peter Rober.
Other titles: Gezinstherapeut zijn. English
Description: First English edition. | Abingdon, Oxon ; New York, NY : Routledge, 2024. |
"First English edition published 2024 by Routledge ... First Dutch edition published by Pelckmans 2023"-- CIP galley. | Includes bibliographical references and index. |
Identifiers: LCCN 2023047204 (print) | LCCN 2023047205 (ebook) | ISBN 9781032602653 (hbk) | ISBN 9781032602677 (pbk) | ISBN 9781003458395 (ebk)
Subjects: LCSH: Family psychotherapy. | Family psychotherapy--Methodology. | Family psychotherapy--Case studies. | Psychotherapist and patient. | Family therapists.
Classification: LCC RC488.5 .R62813 2024 (print) | LCC RC488.5 (ebook) | DDC 616.89/156--dc23/eng/20231220
LC record available at https://lccn.loc.gov/2023047204
LC ebook record available at https://lccn.loc.gov/2023047205

ISBN: 978-1-032-60265-3 (hbk)
ISBN: 978-1-032-60267-7 (pbk)
ISBN: 978-1-003-45839-5 (ebk)

DOI: 10.4324/9781003458395

Typeset in Sabon
by MPS Limited, Dehradun

I became a family therapist at 31
when I graduated
at Leuven University.
But in fact
I have been becoming a family therapist
since my early childhood.

Thank you,
Mom and Dad.
Thank you,
my brothers and my sisters,
for teaching me
most of what I needed to learn
to become a family therapist.

# Contents

# Introduction

## The story of Filip and Zoë

It's the first session. Filip (16 years old) talks cautiously about his withdrawn life, without friends and activities. He often feels lonely and misunderstood. And that got worse last summer when his sister Zoë (19 years old) went to study at the university in Leuven.

Filip: "Yes, I actually miss my sister ..."

He leaves a silence, and it strikes me that he looks sad.

I turn to Zoë: "Do you miss your brother sometimes?"

Zoë says, "Not at all. I have my life and he has his. I have a lot of friends and I'm busy in Leuven."

That touches me because it must be terrible for Filip to hear. *Doesn't Zoë have any connection with him?*

I try again: "But you sometimes think about your brother? Do you worry about him sometimes?" When I hear my own words, I notice that they don't sound right. I hear in my words that according to me she *should* think of him, that she *should be* worried. I realize that I am completely absorbed in Filip's perspective and that I am not showing any real interest in Zoë and in her perspective.

Zoë replies: "To be honest: no, I don't think much about him. I do my own things."

These words strike me: *my own things.*

I say, "Tell me about those things, Zoë ..." and I hear that this question is an appropriate correction to my previous attempts to connect with her. I show genuine interest in Zoë.

DOI: 10.4324/9781003458395-1

Zoë then says that in Leuven she closes herself off from the worries about home.

"Only in this way I can survive," she says. "After all, a lot goes wrong at home. Not only with Filip. What is worse are the tensions between our parents, who hardly speak to each other anymore. And that weighs heavily on Filip, and he closes himself off, like I close myself off in Leuven."

I feel that Zoë is now making contact with her brother, and I see Filip cautiously nodding in agreement. That reassures me and I decide to address the parents.

I say, "Both of you children are trying to shut themselves off from what is happening at home. Tell me how things are going at home."

### What is family therapy?

There is a clear and simple description of what family therapy is: *a therapist talks with a family in which one or more family members are worried about something.* So, in essence, there's nothing magical about family therapy: it involves a series of conversations with families. The challenge for the family therapist lies in the way the family enters: they are in emotional crisis. There is anger, fear, despair, or sadness; sometimes in the open but often covered in silence. And there is no trust: neither in each other, nor in themselves, nor in the world that is hard and cold when things are really bad.

That is the challenge for the family therapist: *how can I start a therapeutic process with these people?* They are not in a state where they can put their best foot forward. Rather, they are afraid and cramped, insecure and angry, cautious, and waiting … and there you are as a family therapist.

The family comes in with their worries and their suffering. The reduction of the suffering of the family is the ultimate goal. In the session, however, the therapist is not primarily focused on problem solving or on healing. Too narrow a focus on alleviating suffering appears to lead to powerlessness and frustration. In the first place, the therapist is focused on promoting the trust between the family members and on the connection between them. A better connection in the session has the effect that the therapeutic interventions work deeper and talking starts to feel good again. Gradually more trust is surfacing, the family members cautiously open up, and healing words can reach deeper to touch the family's sensitive strings. The therapy becomes a corrective emotional experience for the family. The family therapist realizes that these new connections promote the family's own problem-solving resources, and their self-healing powers.

A family therapy session usually starts out cautiously with silences and polite words, but then – as trust is growing – gradually more emotions are evoked in everyone involved, including the therapist. Sadness, pain, anger, fear, despair ... the emotions saturate the session.

The therapist must undergo these emotions him/herself. But unlike the family members, the therapist must remain calm and fulfill his/her role as a therapist. Notwithstanding all the emotions, he/she is expected to sympathize as well as empathize with each of the family members. In that way the therapist contributes to the emergence of a dialogical context in which the unexpected can happen. Because most of the time – in my experience – change is not planned. It happens. At a certain moment. In a certain way. And the therapist may be as surprised as anybody else when it happens. Still, the therapist has contributed to the change. Maybe not so much by what he/she said or did. They probably make a difference especially by being present with the family members: listening, empathizing with the suffering of each family member, trying to understand each family member, seeing each family members' good intentions ... that's an important part of the art of *being a family therapist*. The presence of the family therapist makes it possible for the family members to talk in another way with each other than they do at home: they listen more to each other, they don't lose themselves in escalations, they start to accept their differences ...

In the professional literature, the importance of the therapist's *presence* is highlighted (Hayes & Vinca, 2017). *Presence* is a state of being open to the other, while keeping in touch with oneself. The therapist's attention is focused on the family members, while he/she remains well centered with himself/herself. He/she is constantly trying to find a balance in this, and typically, when he/she thinks he/she has found the right balance, it eludes him/her again. This keeps the therapist busy. Like Sisyphus who is condemned to push the boulder up the hill again and again.

The therapist must set clear goals and have a coherent plan for reaching them. But the goals should in fact not be his/her goals, but the clients'. The difficulty often is that clients are ambivalent about what they want because life is complex and unpredictable. Specifically for family therapy, the challenge is also the diversity in the family in which not all family members think therapy is a good idea. Usually, they have different opinions about the so-called problem. They may even disagree if there is a problem at all.

So the family therapist may have a clear goal and a sound plan to reach that goal. However, the therapist's step-by-step plan is likely to collide with the stubborn dynamics of what happens in the family session, as well as in family life. The family therapist must be flexible enough to responsively modify the carefully thought-out plan considering the continuous new developments and the unforeseen circumstances in the session. The reality of psychotherapy usually is messy (Hill & Norcross, 2023) and in some respects the therapist may be best compared to a blindfolded archer: there may be a clear aim somewhere but the archer can't see it and he/she has to use other senses than his/her vision to orient and find the right general direction of the bulls eye.

### Becoming an effective family therapist

This book should be read against the background of the psychotherapy research that shows that there are therapist effects: psychotherapy is effective, and all bona fide psychotherapy models are about equally effective. But therapists are not equally effective. Some are more effective, and others are less effective. Research shows that effective therapists form strong therapeutic alliances across a wide range of patients (Wampold, 2017). With some patients it is easy to form an alliance: they are motivated to change and they are prepared to work hard. They have a supporting social network, a secure attachment style, and elaborate interpersonal skills. Every therapist can form a strong alliance with these patients. But there are other patients too: not motivated, discouraged, socially isolated, not so talented socially or intellectually, and so on ... These patients are much more of a challenge for therapist, and they make the difference between an effective therapist and a less effective therapist.

In recent years, there have been several books on this issue, focusing on the question what can make a therapist more effective (Castonguay & Hill, 2017). Often the focus is on the skills of the therapist (e.g. Rousmaniere, 2019; Miller & Moyers, 2021) and the therapist's deliberate practice is promoted the royal road for the therapist to improve his/her clinical effectiveness (e.g. Rousmaniere, 2017).

However, in these publications the focus is on individual therapy and the specific effectiveness of the *family therapist* has hardly been considered. Still, family therapy is complex, and particularly the complex alliance in family therapy makes it challenging. So one would expect that the difference between effective therapists and less effective therapists is even more important in family therapy than in individual therapy. As far as I know, we don't have scientific data to corroborate this claim, but based on what we know about the effectiveness of therapist this claim makes sense.

In this book the family therapist's effectiveness will be central, but rather than listing discrete skills the family therapist should master, I will focus on the family therapist in the process: the therapist in the session with the family. I will describe family therapy as a meeting of living persons searching to find ways to share life together for a while. The emphasis is on *being together*. Yes, when I try to describe the specific angle of this book, the language becomes fuzzier and velvety. But let me reassure you, dear reader, in this book I will not go deeper into the dialogical and existential philosophical background of the approach I'm presenting. I have written about this background extensively in the past (e.g. Rober, 2005b; 2017b). The focus of the book will remain practical and down to earth, although its philosophical background will unavoidably marinate my words and saturate my stories.

## Being a family therapist

Being a family therapist is a lifelong learning process of *becoming*, in which the therapist develops further and further into who he/she is. Inspired by the experiential family therapist David Keith (Keith & Paparone, 2017), we can say that there are three stages in the development of a family therapist.

1 *Learning about family therapy*, in which knowledge about families and about family therapy is central.
2 *Learning to do family therapy*, in which learning intervention techniques and following step-by-step treatment protocols are central.
3 *Being a family therapist*, where the person of the family therapist is central. What the therapist has learned in terms of useful knowledge, intervention techniques and protocols is so well practiced that it has been incorporated: it has become part of the therapist's person. To appeal to that knowledge or expertise in the session, it is no longer necessary for the therapist to think about it: it has become intuitive, and the implicit knowledge can guide the therapist's actions without his/her explicit reflection.

This book is about *being a family therapist*. I will summarize the knowledge we have about psychotherapy in general, and about family therapy in particular. I will also dwell on some of the ways in which a therapist can approach a family session. But the emphasis in this book is on the person of the family therapist who is present with the suffering family and tries to be useful and make him/herself redundant.

Part I

# What scientific research can teach us about being an effective therapist

# 1 The effective psychotherapist

Is psychotherapy effective? If so, what makes psychotherapy effective? These are the central questions in this chapter in which we will go over the recent scientific research on psychotherapy. While this book is about family therapy, this chapter has a broader scope: the focus is on psychotherapy in general. We start from the assumption that what applies to psychotherapy in general can also teach us something about family therapy.

## Psychotherapy is overall effective

The research of psychotherapy in recent decades shows that psychotherapy is overall effective (Barkham & Lambert, 2021): a large number of clients benefit from psychotherapy (not all of them). They make significant changes in their lives with the help of a therapist.

Research shows that psychotherapy works well but is certainly not perfect. Not everyone is helped, some clients recover with the help of therapy but relapse later, and some clients (luckily a small minority) get worse (Barkham & Lambert, 2021).

---

### The effect of psychotherapy

Researchers Wampold and Imel (2015) state that psychotherapy has an effect size of .75 to .80. The effect size (in this book we use Cohen $d$ as an index) is a statistical measure with which we can compare different treatments, but what does it mean? An effect size of .80 means that the average person who goes to therapy does better after a while than 79% of the people who did not go to therapy.

The fact that people who go to therapy improve on average does not mean that this improvement can be attributed to the therapy itself: only about 14% of the result of psychotherapy is explained by

---

DOI: 10.4324/9781003458395-3

the psychotherapy itself (Wampold & Imel, 2015). Most of the result of the therapy is the result of factors that have nothing to do with the therapy itself. This concerns characteristics of the client and of his/her environment: for example, the client receives a promotion at work that puts him/her in a better functioning team; the client falls in love and suddenly sees a bright future; the client moves to a larger house with a beautiful garden in which he/she starts a vegetable garden; etc. All these changes in the client's life can have a major impact on his/her psychological well-being. In fact, it has a lot more impact than psychotherapy does.

It is not an entirely new finding that the client's life outside of therapy makes a major contribution to the outcome of psycho-therapy (see e.g. Hubble, Duncan, & Miller, 1999; Bohart & Greaves Wade, 2013), but it remains an observation that is often forgotten in the *evidence-based* climate that dominates mental health care. It is also a finding that should make us think: in my practice as a psychotherapist, how can I best use the client and context factors of my clients in the service of their well-being? This question has been considered before (see e.g. Duncan & Miller, 2000), but it certainly deserves further reflection.

**About the importance of treatment models**

Research also shows that there are hardly differences in effectiveness between different therapeutic treatment models (Barkham & Lambert, 2021). When we talk about treatment models, we refer to the various therapeutic models that are academically anchored; what Wampold calls *bona fide* treatments (Wampold & Imel, 2015). They are theoretically and conceptually developed, and there is good quality empirical research demonstrating their efficacy. Broadly speaking, it concerns (cognitive) behavioral therapeutic, experiential, psychodynamic, and systemic (family and couple therapeutic) models. These models are very different in terms of theory, concepts, and interventions, but these differences do not appear to lead to large and consistent differences in efficacy. These different therapy models are all roughly equally effective (Barkham & Lambert, 2021).

Although there are no differences in their effectiveness, treatment models are important. They are needed for therapy to work. This is evident from research into the factors that make therapy work. For example, there is the meta-analysis of Wampold (2015) in which the relative influence of different therapy factors on the effectiveness of therapy (expressed in effect size) was investigated.

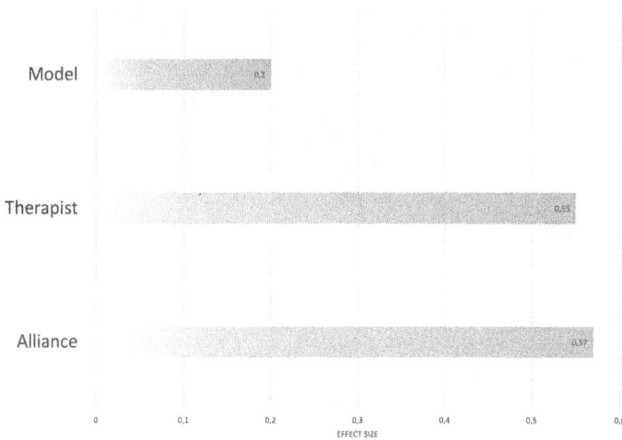

*Figure 1.1* Factors contributing to the effectiveness of psychotherapy.

This diagram shows that the alliance (the therapeutic relationship) and the therapist contribute more to the outcome of psychotherapy than the treatment model does. But the effect of the model is not zero. This seems to indicate: a therapist must have a model if he/she wants to achieve results with psychotherapy, although it may not matter that much which model it is (Barkham & Lambert, 2021).

---

**The therapeutic relationship is crucial**

An effect size of .57 indicates that the *relationship* between the client and the therapist (regardless of the specific therapeutic approach) is very important for the effectiveness of psychotherapy. The quality of that relationship predicts the effect of therapy: if the client feels understood and heard, then there is a good chance that the therapy will work. And vice versa: if the client does not feel understood and heard, there is little chance that the therapy will be helpful.

The main criticism of this finding is that it is based on correlational research, and that a correlation says nothing about the direction of the causality. Is the outcome of the therapy the result of the good therapeutic relationship, or is it the other way around: the therapeutic relationship gets better when the therapy goes well. This is a fair comment and quite a bit of research has been done to look at this connection more closely. Crits-Christoph & Connelly

Gibbons (2021) have listed these studies and they conclude that there is sufficient evidence to speak of a causal relationship between the quality of the therapeutic relationship and the result of psychotherapy. Nevertheless, it will probably be a circular relationship: the good quality of the therapeutic relationship contributes to a good result, and the good evolution of the therapy contributes to a better relationship. In any case, it is important that the therapist in practice deals with the therapeutic relationship with care and dedication (Crits-Christoph & Connelly Gibbons, 2021).

There is a lot of research that can teach us what the ingredients of a good therapeutic relationship must be in order for it to work. These are the most important elements as they emerge from the research of Wampold & Imel (2015): therapist-client collaboration, empathy, affirmation of the client (also called *acceptance*), and authenticity of the therapist (also called *congruence*).

We can show the relative importance of these relationship characteristics for the effectiveness of psychotherapy as follows:

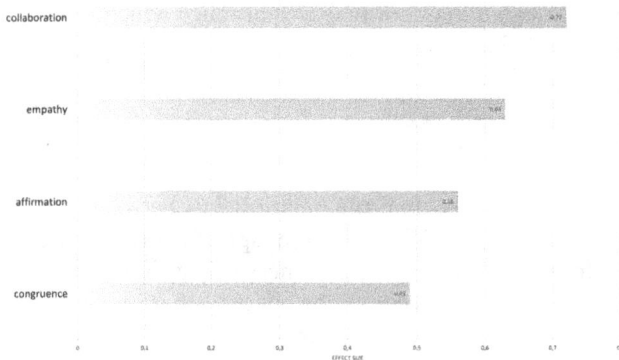

*Figure 1.2* Factors contributing to a good therapeutic alliance.

From this diagram we can learn a lot about the ways in which a therapeutic relationship can best be shaped. An effective therapeutic relationship is a collaborative relationship, in which the therapist is really present as a human being and in which he/she empathizes with the client. The therapist is also focused on affirming the client by seeing his/her commitment and good intentions, and by paying attention to the client's own growth potentials and healing powers.

**Empirical affirmation of Rogers' vision**

It is remarkable how contemporary psychotherapy research largely agrees with Carl Rogers (1902–1987) in his view of therapy. After all, Rogers had put forward three necessary conditions for therapeutic change: empathy, authenticity, and acceptance. The importance of these three conditions is now also confirmed by the empirical research. Rogers did say that those conditions were not only *necessary*, but also *sufficient* (if those conditions are met, therapeutic change will automatically follow, Rogers claimed). This last point is not confirmed by research, because studies show that the therapeutic relationship is very important, but it also shows that more than just a good therapeutic relationship is needed to achieve therapeutic change. For example, a therapeutic treatment model is also needed. Furthermore, the therapeutic relationship needs also to be a working alliance: it must be a collaborative relationship in which there is an agreement between therapist and client about the purpose of the therapy, and about the general method that one will follow.

## The therapist in outcome research

Wampold's research (2015) also shows that, although there are hardly any differences in effectiveness between models (effect size 0.20), there are large differences in effectiveness between therapists (effect size 0.55). This suggests that some therapists achieve better outcomes than other therapists, regardless of the model they use (Castonguay & Hill, 2017; Wampold & Owens, 2021). So there are effective behavioral therapists, and less effective behavioral therapists. There are effective psychodynamic therapists and less effective psychodynamic therapists. Ditto for experiential therapists and family therapists. It is also clear that the difference in effectiveness cannot be explained by the characteristics of the clients, nor by the Interaction effects of the client and therapist. No, this is about therapists who consistently achieve better results than others over a range of clients and diagnoses. In the scientific literature this is called *therapist effects* (Baldwin & Imel, 2013; Barkham et al., 2017; Johns, Barkham, Kellett, & Saxon, 2019; Wampold & Owens, 2021). Overall, we know that the effect of the therapist is greater if the client's problems are more severe (Johns et al., 2019). With more difficult clients, the difference between a good therapist and a bad one comes to the fore.

**Diagnosis-treatment combination**

The fact that there are important differences in effectiveness between different therapists shows that thinking in terms of the diagnosis-treatment combination (DBC) is scientifically outdated. In contrast to the medical science, the challenge for our field is not to find a good combination between a diagnosis on the one hand and a treatment on the other. In psychotherapy being effective is much more than just administering the appropriate treatment. Psychotherapy research tells us that effective psychotherapy mainly depends on the *relationship between the therapist and the client*, rather than on the treatment itself. And yes, some therapists are better at forming such relationships than other therapists.

The difference in effectiveness between therapists can be represented in the form of a bell curve:

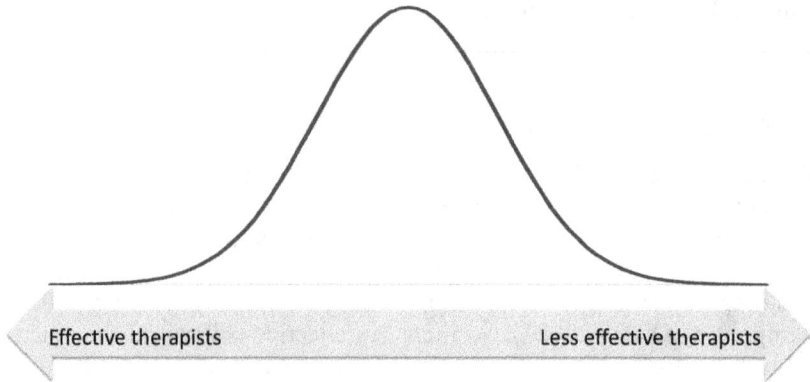

Effective therapists                    Less effective therapists

*Figure 1.3* The bell curve of the effectiveness of psychotherapists.

This image shows the different therapists from more to less effective. It is clear that most therapists are situated somewhere in the middle of the bell curve: they are sometimes more effective, and sometimes less effective. In addition, the curve depicts that some therapists are consistently less effective (right) and others are consistently very effective (left).

The observation that there are differences in effectiveness between therapists has led to a new focus on the therapist in psychotherapy research (Castonguay & Hill, 2017). Researchers started to focus on the group of the most effective therapists, with the question: "What makes these therapists so effective?" They started to search for the more or less stable characteristics of effective therapists.

This research is very important. It not only helps us to better understand what makes psychotherapy effective, but it can also help us improve the training of therapists: What should we teach young therapists so that they can become more effective? Apparently, teaching treatment models, concepts, and intervention techniques is less important than we previously thought. But what is important?

### Characteristics of effective therapists that are not related to the result of therapy

Not all characteristics of therapists are important. For example, it has been found that most objective characteristics of therapists (e.g. age, gender, prior education, etc.) do not have a consistent influence on the effectiveness of therapists (Beutler et al., 2004; Wampold & Owens, 2021). A female therapist is no better than a male one. An older therapist is no better than a younger one. Etc.

But it is all complex. For one thing, it turns out that age does not matter that much in itself, but age difference with the client may (Beutler et al., 2004). The same applies to the ethnic identity of the therapist: therapists of European, African, or Asian origin are equally effective, but similarity in ethnicity between therapist and client may benefit the result of therapy (Beutler et al., 2004; Wampold & Owens, 2021).

Furthermore, there is a great deal of uncertainty about how important *professional experience* is for the effectiveness of the therapist. Therapists themselves assume that they become more effective the more experienced they are (Orlinsky & Rønnestad, 2005). Perhaps most laymen would agree that this is an obvious assumption. However, contrary to what is taken as obvious, research does not unequivocally indicate that experienced therapists are more effective than inexperienced therapists (eg. Beutler et al., 2004; Wampold & Owens, 2021; Goldberg et al., 2016). It is complex. Research shows that more experienced therapists have less *drop-out* of clients (Goldberg et al., 2016). Furthermore, research suggests that we should not see the concept of professional experience as the *quantity* of the therapist's professional experience (how many years of experience), but that it makes more sense to look at the *quality* of the experience: What kind of professional experience does the therapist have? For example, a review study of the available research indicates that the amount of contact with clients (rather than the experience with specific interventions) would be important for the effectiveness of therapists (Beutler et al., 2004), especially when it comes to treating more complex cases (Beutler, Bongar, & Shurkin, 1998). In the same vein, Wampold and

Imel (2015) state on the basis of the meta-analysis of Webb, DeRubeis, and Barber (2010) that there is no correlation between the competence of the therapist and the therapy outcome when it comes to specific competencies that have to do with specific treatments or interventions. When it comes to non-specific competencies (e.g. the ability to form a warm therapeutic relationship), there is a connection with the outcome of therapy: the more experience therapists have with forming therapeutic relationships (with a wide variety of clients) the better the outcomes they achieve in their therapeutic work.

**Therapeutic characteristics that are predictive of the outcome of therapy**

There is gradually more research into the characteristics of effective therapists, but this field of research is rather new, and much further research is needed (Wampold & Owens, 2021). An overview of the research until now shows that characteristics of therapists that deal with their life outside of therapy (e.g. social skills in private life, attitudes in personal life) do not seem to be directly related to the result of therapy (Heinonen & Nissen-Lie, 2020). Therapist characteristics that are predictive of effective psychotherapy are mainly about professional characteristics. Some characteristics that relate to what the therapist does during the session and how he/she deals with the challenges that arise there appear to correlate well with the result of the therapy (Heinonen & Nissen-Lie, 2020).

There is sufficient research evidence to say that these are the characteristics of effective therapists (Norcross & Lambert, 2019; Wampold & Owens, 2021):

1 *An effective therapist is focused on building a good working relationship.* He/she makes an effort to achieve a good working relationship with the clients (Tryon, Birch, & Verkuilen, 2019). This means, among other things, that effective therapists invite the client to actively give direction to the process, that they are focused on the client's concerns, that they make agreements with their client about the purpose of the therapy, that they consult with the client about important choices that need to be made, that they ask for feedback from their client and take this feedback into account as much as possible, and so on. Forcing or pressuring clients is never a good idea. Expecting the client to be docile and compliant does not contribute to the therapist's effectiveness either. The therapist and the client working together in a respectful way, each from his/her own role is best; this is also evident from the research by Wampold (2015) to which we referred above. Of all factors, collaboration is most strongly linked to a good result of therapy (effect size 0.72).

*An effective therapist possesses the interpersonal qualities to build a warm and empathetic relationship of trust* (Anderson, Ogles, Lambert, & Vermeersch, 2009; Anderson & Hill, 2017; Schöttke, Flückiger, Goldberg, Eversman, & Lange, 2017). In the scientific literature one speaks of *facilitative interpersonal skills* (FIS). These skills are therapist qualities such as verbal and emotional expressiveness, being able to read the client's emotions well and deal with them constructively, being hopeful and warm, being focused on what the client experiences as a problem, being able to tolerate criticism and deal with it constructively, etc.

2 An important therapist characteristic that fits in with this is *empathy*. There is a lot of research that shows that empathy is important for the outcome of psychotherapy (Elliott, Bohart, Watson, & Murphy, 2019). It is one of the most potent predictors of client progress in psychotherapy. This means that an effective therapist must be focused on understanding the client's experiences, thoughts, and feelings, and on attuning to the client. The therapist's empathy offers the client an authentic nonjudgmental connection with the therapist that invites the client to reflect further on his/her own experiences, to seek words for an authentic story about these experiences, and to share this story with the therapist, who in turn listens empathetically to what the client recounts.

---

### Difficult clients

The difference between effective and less effective therapists is most acute among difficult clients. This may concern clients with a more serious diagnosis (e.g. a complex trauma, instead of a simple trauma), or clients with whom it is more difficult to build a good collaborative relationship (e.g. because they are not motivated, or are suspicious, critical, silent). We know this from a lot of research (e.g. Johns et al., 2019; Barkham & Lambert, 2021). The most important thing appears to be that the therapist manages to use his/her negative feelings towards the client (frustration, irritation, boredom, etc.) constructively in his/her therapeutic actions (Wolf, Goldfried, & Muran, 2017).

Broadly speaking, one could say that the client can present the therapist with challenges in two ways: firstly, by withdrawing (keeping quiet, keeping distance, etc.); secondly by being confrontational (criticizing, expressing displeasure, etc.). The way in which the therapist deals with these difficult interpersonal challenges is crucial for building a good therapeutic relationship, especially in family therapy where the therapeutic relationship is more complex than in individual therapy (see chapter 2). In addition, the way in which the therapist deals with his/her own emotions is of great importance (see chapter 6) and it is often primarily important that the therapist protects the therapeutic relationship against his/her own difficult emotions (irritation, boredom, fear, etc.). As I will explain in chapter 6, in some cases it is even possible for the therapist to find a way to make those difficult emotions contribute to useful interventions. This illustrates that the therapist's interpersonal skills are critical (Anderson et al., 2009; Anderson & Hill, 2017).

3 *The effective therapist is able to be present with the client in an accepting and hopeful way.* This means that the therapist does not judge the client, but understands his/her experiences as authentic, human experiences (Farber, Suzuki, & Lynch, 2019). Furthermore, he/she sees and acknowledge the client's efforts and attempts to make life better and does this without denying or minimizing the client's suffering. The therapist is realistically hopeful that the therapy can lead to improvement, even if the client him/herself has little hope (Constantino, Vîslă, Coyne, & Boswell, 2019). The effective therapist has a positive and humane view of the client's suffering, as well as a positive and humane explanation for why therapy can be useful (Wampold, 2017).

4 *The effective therapist is constantly questioning him/herself as a professional, in a context of self-confidence and being gentle with oneself.* In the scientific literature this is called *professional self-doubt* (Nissen-Lie et al., 2017), and it is stated that this presupposes a certain *modesty* or even *humility* (Heinonen & Nissen-Lie, 2020). It turns out that the extent to which a therapist questions him/herself as a therapist is related to a good therapy outcome (Wampold, 2017). Such questioning is sometimes called *self-reflection* or *self-supervision* (Rober, 2021). It is important that the therapist has sufficient self-confidence and that he/she has a positive self-image overall. "Love yourself as a person, doubt yourself as a therapist", say Nissen-Lie and her colleagues (Nissen-Lie et al., 2017): the therapist must have enough self-confidence to dare to look critically at him/herself and to wonder whether he/she is doing well in his/her attempts to help the client.

5 *The effective therapist works systematically with the client's feedback.* The client's feedback is useful to build a good working relationship and to build a safe relationship of trust (Lambert, Whipple, & Kleinstäuber, 2019). Furthermore, the feedback from the client is also an important

factor in the therapist's self-reflections because that feedback shows the effect of the therapist's efforts. Client feedback appears to be of greatest use if the therapeutic process does not go well (Lambert, et al., 2019): it makes the therapist aware that things are not working. This is important as research shows that therapists are overconfident in the evaluation of their own effectiveness (Walfish et al., 2012). Client feedback can notify the therapist about what is not optimal in the eyes of the client. In some cases, it also gives suggestions on how things can be improved. This is not only about collecting client feedback by the therapist, but certainly also about reflecting with the client about this feedback with the intention of tailoring the therapy to the client's needs as much as possible. In addition, it is an important challenge for the therapist that he/she deals with the feedback given by the client in a constructive, non-defensive way, and that he/she can enter an open dialogue with the client about the feedback. Knowing that client feedback is especially useful when it is critical and detailed, it is often not self-evident for the therapist to listen openly and non-defensively to the client's concerns about the session. In chapter 7 we will consider the family therapist's feedback orientation in extenso.

Perhaps we can summarize the characteristics of effective therapists in one sentence: effective therapists succeed in building a good therapeutic relationship with many different clients, including challenging or difficult clients (Wampold, Baldwin, Holtforth & Imel, 2017). In other words, the therapeutic relationship is the crucial concern of the effective therapist.

An important point in this context is that about all the insights about the importance of the therapist characteristics for the effectiveness of therapy that are summarized in this chapter are largely based on research done on individual therapists. As far as I know, no specific research has yet been done on the importance of the family therapist in the therapeutic process. Is there reason to believe that it would be different in family therapy than in individual therapy? Some authors argue that family therapy is more complex and that, even more than in individual therapy, the therapist's skills will make a difference in the efficacy of the therapy (Karam & Blow, 2023). I will assume in this book that what emerges from research for individual therapy (i.e. that the specific therapist makes an important difference in the effectiveness of therapy) also applies to family therapy. I will also assume that this is mainly (but not exclusively) due to the ability of the family therapist to build a good alliance with many different families.

From the next chapter on, and in the rest of the book, I will focus on family therapy and on the way the complexity of the therapeutic relationship in family therapy affects the therapist in the session. I will also consider ways in which the therapist can deal with this complexity and offer case stories as illustration. Now and again, but not very often, I will refer to individual therapy, but I will do so mainly to highlight the specificity of family therapy.

# 2 The complex alliance in family therapy

## Stan and his family

I remember the first time I met a family in therapy. It must have been in 1987 or 1988, and I had graduated as a clinical child psychologist, but I had not yet started my training as a family therapist. A mother and two sons (Stan, 16, and Louis, 13 years old) were waiting for me to start the session. As I was taught by my psychotherapy professor (an individual therapist) I asked them, "How can I help you?" I made sure to make eye contact with the three family members in turn, because I wanted them to know that I was addressing each of them.

Mother replied and began to talk about her concerns. She was particularly concerned about 16-year-old Stan, who had skipped a few classes and was questioned by the police last week because of possession of cannabis. Mother explained how she had lived alone with her two children after their father left her about 12 years ago. She had to combine a full-time job as a nurse with raising two boys, which was not easy. Fortunately, she had some help from her mother who was also alone after divorcing her husband (mother's father, the children's grandfather). And so on. I listened carefully, nodded occasionally, and at appropriate times said "mmm" and "I understand".

When Mom finished her story, I turned to Stan and asked him, "Stan, how can I help you?"

Stan's answer was short: "Who says I need help?"

He looked at his mother defiantly.

This was a hint for mother.

She turned to Stan and said, "Of course you need help. Look at how things are going. Your life is a mess, as is your bedroom. You refuse to go to school and now you've been arrested by the police ..."

DOI: 10.4324/9781003458395-4

Stan rolled his eyes and said, "I wasn't arrested."

"Yes, you were," mother said, "and they called me, and I got you out of jail."

"I've never been in jail!" cried Stan, looking away.

Louis turned to his mother and tried to calm her down.

"Mama, please, don't overdo it. He wasn't in jail. He was only questioned by the police."

"You're both against me. Ungrateful pigs." Mother sighed.

The session went on for another 25 minutes and it was a disaster. I was overwhelmed by the power of conflict dynamics in the family. I didn't know what to do. At first, I tried to get some structure into the session, and I called on everyone to listen to each other and to not interrupt each other, but to no avail. And then I gave up. I didn't do anything anymore. I just let it happen. I was defeated.

The family did not show up for a second session.

Looking back on the session with this family, I feel some shame and especially remorse. I should have helped this family better. I wonder how Stan's life is going now (he must be in his fifties by now). But there is more than shame and remorse. I also feel happy because I realize how much I've learned. I'm not the therapist I used to be. Among other things, I learned how to establish a good therapeutic relationship with families. Not that it always works out, but it works much better than it did then.

### The therapeutic relationship

In chapter 1, I explained that research on psychotherapy teaches us that psychotherapy often works well (Barkham & Lambert, 2021). It also teaches us that the effect of psychotherapy can largely be explained by the quality of the therapeutic relationship (Norcross & Lambert, 2018).

---

**The link between the therapeutic alliance and the *outcome* of family therapy**

In chapter 1, I referred to the meta-analysis of Wampold & Imel (2015) where they found an effect size of 0.57. Specifically for family therapy, a meta-analysis by Friedlander, Escudero, Welmers-van der Poll, & Heatherington (2018) found a stronger link between alliance and outcome (effect size 0.62). It seems that in family therapy, the therapeutic relationship is even more important than in individual therapy.

But what does that mean, "the quality of the therapeutic relationship"? What characteristics must a therapeutic relationship have in order to be judged *as good*? In the previous chapter, referring to Wampold's research, I already pointed out the importance of the collaborative relationship, empathy, authenticity, and validation (Wampold & Imel, 2015). Overall, we can also say that the therapeutic relationship must be tailored to the unique client (Norcross & Lambert, 2019). It is tailor-made, not ready-to-wear. With one client it should be more *this*, in the other more *that*, depending on the characteristics of the person (rather than the diagnosis). Considering the therapeutic relationship, two perspectives are especially important:

1  *The working alliance*: therapist and client must collaborate, and there must be consensus between therapist and client about the purpose of the therapy. This consensus can be created by talking to the client about the requests for help, the expectations, the concerns, and so on. The therapist then tries to orient the therapeutic process as much as possible in the direction that the client wants to take. This is how a *working alliance* is formed. There appears to be a link between the quality of the working relationship and the result of the therapy (Gelso, Kivlighan, & Markin, 2019).
2  *The relationship of trust*: a good quality relationship of trust must grow between the therapist and the client. The client sometimes starts the therapy a bit anxious and suspicious ("Will the therapist understand me?", "Will the therapist judge me?", "Will the therapist give me an embarrassing diagnosis?", etc.). If the client during the session begins to feel understood and accepted by the therapist (rather than assessed or labeled), trust will grow, and the client will feel safer to engage in therapy. To make such a relationship of trust possible, the therapist must identify with the client (*I am like you*), without losing the therapist's own position (*I am a therapist, and you are a client*). He/she must empathize with the client's experiences, and still to a certain extent remain an outsider. It's a balance (Miller & Moyers, 2021).

In addition, the therapist must also be congruent (Rogers, 1957): the empathy must be authentic and genuine (Miller & Moyers, 2021). One sometimes also speaks of the *real relationship*, referring to a therapeutic relationship that is realistic (not fraught with all kinds of fears and desires) and that is real (authentic) (Gelso et al., 2019). It refers to the therapeutic relationship from person to person that has not been clouded or distorted by transference or projections of the client. There appears to be a link between the quality of the *real relationship* and the result of the therapy, and that link is stronger than the link between the working alliance and the result of the therapy (Gelso et al., 2019).

The therapist must not only be authentically empathetic, he/she must also accept the client. Some speak of the importance of *affirming* or *validating* the client. A hopeful and positive view of the therapist of the client contributes to a good therapy result (Farber et al., 2019). Rogers (1957) even spoke of *unconditional positive regard* as a condition for successful therapy. However, it is questionable to what extent *unconditional* acceptance within psychotherapy is possible. After all, psychotherapy is pre-eminently an enterprise that is subject to conditions (to name one example: the client must pay the therapist). Maybe unconditional acceptance can only be expected from a parent towards his/her child (and even then). In this sense, it is perhaps not surprising that a therapeutic relationship is often referred to as an attachment relationship. The father of attachment theory John Bowlby (1988) suggested that a psychotherapist can be seen as a kind of attachment figure. After all, a therapist – like a mother or a father – should be a reliable and sensitive person (what Bowlby called a *secure base*) who helps the client in his/her exploration of the world, and who is present at times when the client encounters difficulties.

---

**Parents as secure attachment figures**

Thomas (4 years old) goes with his parents to the playground and sees a child on the swing. Thomas looks intensely at the child and is intrigued.

Father notices this and asks, "Do you also feel like going on the swing?"

Thomas nods.

"Fine," father says. "A swing is a lot of fun."

Mother follows the conversation between father and son and when they step to the swing she says: "Be careful, Thomas, hold on tight with both hands."

Thomas is a bit insecure but says, "Yes, mommy."

Father goes to the swing with Thomas. He puts Thomas on the chair and starts rocking softly, but he holds Thomas with both hands so that he certainly can't fall off.

Thomas doesn't like it much at first and he's a bit scared, but gradually he starts to enjoy the soft rocking.

"Hold on tight with both hands," father says, "I'll stay here with you but I'm going to let you go, ok?"

> Thomas nods and father let's go of the swing and gives Thomas a gentle nudge.
>
> Thomas now holds on to the ropes with his hands and rocks softly.
>
> Father says, "You see, you can do it all by yourself."
>
> Thomas holds himself a bit convulsively because he is insecure, but when he hears father's words, he is proud.
>
> He shouts to his mom who is sitting on a bench a little further away: "Look mom, I can do it all by myself."
>
> At some point, it's enough. Thomas asks father to help him off the swing.
>
> Father does so and Thomas runs to his mother. When he comes to her, she already has her arms open to hug him.
>
> "You're a big boy," mother says.
>
> "It was fun," says Thomas, who is enjoying the embrace and is proud of what he has accomplished.

Unlike a real mother and father, the therapist is a *temporary* attachment figure (e.g. Farber, Lippert, & Nevas, 1995; Dozier & Tyrrell, 1998): the client will have to let go of the therapist at the end of the therapy and move on with his/her life alone. In family therapy, the idea of the therapist as a temporary attachment figure was introduced by John Byng-Hall (1995). In line with attachment thinking, he stated that the therapist has 2 functions as a safe haven: a protective function and an exploratory function.

1 *Protective function*: identifying and empathizing with dangers and conflicts and providing security and comfort. This corresponds to the traditional mother role: dealing firmly and warmly with difficult things in the family, and doing what needs to be done to provide safety (so certainly not denying or ignoring the dangers and conflicts, because that creates a feeling of insecurity).
2 *Exploratory function*: Within the safety of the protective therapist role, the therapist also encourages family members to explore and try new things. The therapist encourages the family members to go further than they have been so far. Together with the family members the therapist is curious and fascinated by the unknown. He/she also believes in the ability of the family members to discover new things or try new roles. In this position, the therapist has more of the traditional father role.

For a therapeutic relationship to be a real secure base for the family members, the therapist must take on both roles: sometimes one, sometimes the other, and often both simultaneously, as parents do. They are the safe haven where the ship can dock. The ship can then be repaired if necessary, or new supplies can be stored or there is time for rest. And then it's time to leave the port to explore the world further.

### The therapeutic relationship in family therapy

In family therapy, the therapeutic relationship is more complex than in individual therapy. After all, in family therapy we have several clients at the same time. The family therapist must build a relationship of trust with each of these clients. Furthermore, the therapist must develop a good working alliance with the family members around some kind of a joint resolution to bring the therapy to a successful conclusion.

Myrna Friedlander and Valentin Escudero have tried to map the complex therapeutic relationship in family therapy in their various publications (e.g. Friedlander, Escudero, & Heatherington, 2006; Escudero & Friedlander, 2017; Friedlander et al., 2018). They emphasize that the therapist must build a relationship of trust with each of the family members, but that trust must also grow *between the family members*. If there is too much distrust between the family members, this can – no matter how good the relationship of trust with the therapist – lead to a situation in which the family members are mainly concerned with protecting themselves (e.g. by remaining silent, by being sarcastic, by attacking the other, etc.) so that the therapeutic process is impeded.

Overall, we can say that the family therapist faces 3 challenges:

- Building a *working alliance* with the family.
- Establishing a relationship of *trust with each of the family members*.
- Stimulating a *relationship of trust between family members*.

We will now delve deeper into each of these challenges.

---

### The ultimate goal of family therapy

In the beginning of a family therapy, the family therapist is mainly focused on connecting with each of the family members and on building the working alliance with the family as a whole.

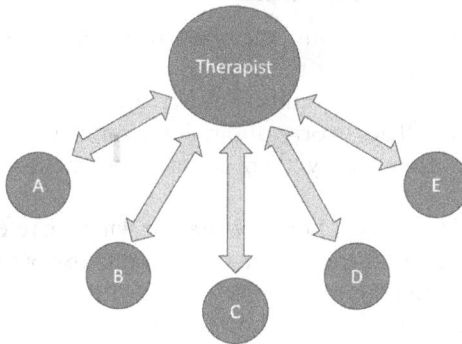

*Figure 2.1* The alliance with each family member.

Only in the second instance – when the therapist has made a first connection with each family member individually, when the working relationship is starting to take form, and when the family members gain some confidence in the therapist – the focus of the family therapist gradually moves to dealing with the relationships between the family members, and trying to optimize the connections between them. The family therapist has specific techniques for this (e.g. *enactment*, see Rober, 2017b).

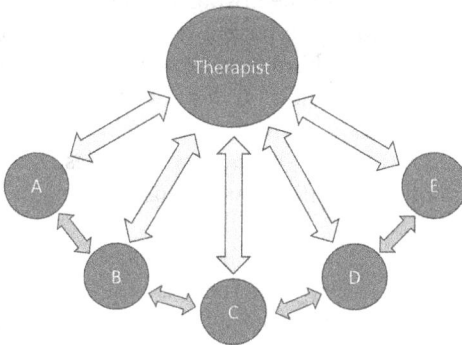

*Figure 2.2* Also the alliance between family members.

This attention to the relationships between family members is in line with the central aim of the family therapist: to promote the exchange between the family members, so that there is more connection in the family, and therefore more safety and comfort.

### The working alliance with the family

It is very exceptional that family members who come to therapy together agree on what the purpose of the therapy is. Usually it is the parents (or one of the parents – in our culture often the mother) who think that therapy is necessary. They worry about something, and they assume that therapy can help them. They then contact the therapist for an initial interview.

Byng-Hall (1995) speaks of the *doorkeeper* when he refers to the person in the family who takes the initiative to go to therapy because that person invites an outsider (the therapist) into the intimate world of the family. As mentioned, it is usually parents who take on the role of doorkeeper. The children rarely take the initiative to go into family therapy. Usually they come along to family therapy, often without knowing what therapy is or without having any idea how therapy might be useful to them. De Shazer (1988) describes such family members as *visitors*. They are present in the session, but they do not really want anything. They are on a visit: they are polite, they look around, and they wait. Besides the visitors, there may be other family members who have been forced to come along to the family therapy against their will. Friedlander et al. (2006) speak in this context of *therapy hostages*: they do not want therapy at all but have been pressured to participate.

The therapist must build a good working alliance with the doorkeepers, as well as with the visitors and the hostages. To this end, it is not necessary for the members of the family to have a clearly formulated common goal. It is important that the family members have a shared *sense of purpose* (Friedlander et al., 2006): a common desire to talk together about what is difficult in the family, and a desire to make it better for everyone in the family. Research shows that in successful therapies, this *shared sense of purpose* in the family gradually strengthens over the course of therapy (Friedlander et al., 2018).

Building a working alliance with a doorkeeper is usually not difficult. The doorkeepers want therapy: in the past they may have made many attempts to deal with their concerns and fears, they may have tried different things to change what is going wrong, but all their efforts have failed. Often the doorkeepers are at their wits' end. That's why they contacted the family therapist. When they finally meet the therapist, they are eager to tell their story. It doesn't take much effort for the therapist to hear from the doorkeepers what their main worries and concerns are.

With the visitors and the hostages, it's completely different. Especially at the start of a family therapy, they are the big challenge for the therapist. They don't really want therapy, or they don't know if they want it yet.

Maybe it's a boy who doesn't understand why dad is so disappointed that he's punished so often at school. Or it could be a young girl who is convinced that there is nothing wrong with her eating, although she refuses to eat most food. Or an adolescent who conflicts with his parents and who resists their decisions or demands. Or a young boy who is worried about his mother's alcohol abuse and doesn't understand why his parents don't say anything about it to the therapist, while they keep on complaining about his truancy at school. There may be hundreds of reasons why family members who come along to the session are not eager to really get involved in therapy.

It is usually not a good idea for the therapist to try to motivate or convince a visitor or a hostage with arguments that therapy can be useful. It often leads to increased distrust, because in this way, the therapist would take the position of the parents who have already tried to convince the child of the importance of therapy. The therapist then would act as an accomplice of the parents, and the child/young person would probably treat him/her as he/she treats his/her parents (suspicious, keeping distance, etc.).

---

**Worries Questionnaire** (free download on www. intherapytogether.com)

For the first session, I send the family members a Worries Questionnaire (see attachment 1) via email, asking that each of the family members fill it out and email it back (Rober, 2017b). The Worries Questionnaire is specifically designed to deal with the complex alliance in family therapy.

In the questionnaire, the family members are first asked who they think is most concerned in the family. In other words, they are asked to indicate who they think is the doorkeeper. Very often – not always – the parents (and especially the mother) are referred to as the most concerned. We then ask what they think the most concerned family member is most worried about.

In the second part of the questionnaire, the family members are asked to indicate how worried they themselves are, and what they are concerned about. Visitors will often indicate that they are not so worried, or that they are worried about something completely different from what the most concerned family member is worried about. Often hostages do not complete the questionnaire.

By systematically administering these Worries Questionnaires before the first interview, the family therapist gets a fairly reliable indication of the different ways in which the different family members look at family therapy even before he/she starts the session. In this way, the family therapist already has an idea before the first session of who in the family is the doorkeeper, and who the visitors and hostages possibly are.

There are three crucial things the therapist must do to build a working relationship:

1 *The therapist listens to the concerns of each of the family members.* By the end of the first session, all family members should have had a chance to talk about their concerns.
2 *The therapist is empathetic to the suffering of each of the family members,* so that each of the family members feels understood in what weighs heavily on him/her. Suffering is the emotional weight of a worry. In this sense, it is very important that the therapist tries to understand how the family member is suffering and what more abstract sensitive strings are vibrating in every concern expressed by the family members. Here, the family therapist must rely on his/her sensitivity and responsiveness as a temporary attachment figure. In this way, the therapist shows that he/she is available as an attachment figure to every family member, and not only to the parents who can explain it well, who have a better command of the appropriate language and who have more authority as adults.

### Existential themes

The focus on the suffering of the different family members brings the therapist into contact with the existential themes that are always implicitly present. It is often – in one form or another – about the four themes that Yalom puts forward in his book *Existential Psychotherapy* (1980): death, freedom, loneliness, and meaninglessness. The focus of the therapist is therefore not on diagnoses, syndromes, and symptoms, but on the deeper experience of each family member and how the concerns in the family are connected to sensitive strings in those essential layers of being human.

By showing interest as a therapist in the suffering, and in the humanity of the various family members, the session can become a real *I-thou* encounter (Buber, 1923), also for the family members themselves (see Rober, 2017b).

3 *The therapist acknowledges* the efforts of each of the family members to deal with the suffering in the family. In that way *each of* the family members feels that the therapist sees their commitment to the family and their attempts to help the family survive. Worries are related to suffering (difficult and painful emotions), but also to commitment: each family member will make attempts in his/her own way to overcome the worries he/she experiences. Often – especially with children and young people – it is about more tacit attempts to help, so that the commitment is often not seen by the other family members. It can even involve symbolic or ritual actions that are more likely to fit into a magical or obsessive-compulsive thinking. It is up to the therapist to notice and acknowledge this commitment – even if it is implicit or ritual.

It is easier to build a working relationship with the family members who are more concerned and who chose to go to therapy themselves (the doorkeepers) than with the hostages who only come along because they have been pressured. And it is tempting for the family therapist to choose the path of least resistance and first make contact with the one who is most worried, and most motivated to start family therapy. However, it is better to resist that temptation.

It is often a good idea to make contact with the hostage as soon as possible in the first session (even if he/she often does not want that contact and explicitly avoids it). The first step is for the therapist to show that he/she accepts that the hostage does not want therapy but has only come along under more or less pressure from the parents. In order to connect with the hostage, it makes more sense to talk about the pressure put on him/her than about the good reasons the doorkeeper has to want therapy. If the hostage feels that the therapist really accepts that he/she does not want therapy, a first empathic contact arises: the visitor expected that the therapist – like the parents – would argue for the importance of therapy or put further pressure on him/her to engage in therapy, but the opposite happens: the therapist shows understanding for the hostage who does not want therapy. This surprises the hostage and that sometimes sets the door ajar. If the therapist then goes on and does not start talking about the parents' complaints but shows authentic interest in the hostage ("who are you?", "what is important for you?", "what do you do that makes you happy?", etc.), something may happen that makes the hostage expose something of him/herself. As the contact grows cautiously, there may also be space after a while in which the hostage dares to show something about his/her own worries (which are probably different from those of the parents), his/her suffering, or his/her commitment to the family. The therapist must notice this (possibly it will be more implicit in the beginning) and the therapist must respond appropriately to this (e.g. "I know you don't want therapy and that's ok, but I hear that at times you feel lonely in the family. What do you do when you feel lonely?"). Usually, this first contact with the hostage works best if the therapist focuses in his/her questions on actions ("what do you do?"), rather than on emotions ("what do you feel?").

The first challenge for the therapist is therefore to make empathetic contact with the family members who least want therapy (the visitors and especially the hostages). That is why he/she has to slow down the doorkeepers, even if they are poised to tell their story, to express their concerns, and to make it clear that they have made a great effort to overcome the difficulties. Making contact with the hostages is especially difficult as most hostages are suspicious and try to keep the therapist at bay. However, it becomes even more difficult when the therapist gives space to the story of the doorkeepers before making contact with the hostage. The story of the doorkeepers is often incriminating for the hostage and will probably make him/her even more defensive and closed.

In summary, we can say that these central questions give the therapist direction in the first contact with the different family members:

1  Who are you?
2  What are you worried about?
3  What is your suffering? (How does this worry weigh on you emotion-ally?)
4  What is your commitment in the family? (How do you want to contribute to a pleasant family life?)

These questions are in the back of the therapist's head during the first session, but it is usually not a good idea to formulate them in this way towards the family members. These questions should be integrated in the warm and accepting way the therapist connects with each of the family members. It is usually best to come up with an appropriate formulation in the living contact with each family member. These four questions of the therapist should be tailored to each specific family member, and by considering each of these questions with each family member, the therapist will establish a good working relationship. In doing so, the therapist listens to the various worries, he/she is empathetic to the suffering, and he/she acknowledges the commitment of each family member. That is the essence of what the therapist has to do in the first session. Usually, a complex picture of a family starts to emerge of the different worries that live in a family, of the suffering of each of the family members and of a faint shared commitment to make living together in the family better for everyone (and especially for those who suffer the most). This is what one might call a *shared sense of purpose* (Friedlander et al., 2006).

**Building a relationship of trust with each of the family members**

To build a working alliance with the various family members, trust must grow between the family members and the therapist. This is very important. After all, sometimes family therapy scares off family members. They may have had counselling sessions in the past that did not go well (with another therapist, with the general practitioner, with a teacher, etc.). Or they have noticed that, when talking at home about what is difficult in the family, it often leads to conflicts, to deep sadness or despair on the part of one of the family members. Going to therapy then feels threatening and the family member will be very hesitant to engage in the sessions. Based on experiences from the past, there is mainly distrust of the therapy. Often this distrust is stronger with a hostage than with a doorkeeper. The more distrust there is, the more the family member may be tempted to provide security himself/herself: by remaining silent, denying, counterattacking, etc. This search for security can make the therapist aware that there is a lot of hesitation on the part of that family member. Rather than verbally reassuring the family member, the therapist should be interested and empathetic about the good reasons of the family member in question to hesitate (Rober, 2017b).

---

**Safety in the session**

The therapeutic session is a place in which family members share stories about their lives and their experiences with the therapist (Friedlander et al., 2006). However, a session doesn't always feel safe for the client, because maybe the therapist isn't going to understand them, or maybe he/she is going to judge them, or maybe he/she is going to think they're "crazy", and so on. Another source of possible insecurity is the other family members: they too may not understand, they may minimize, they may judge, etc. The safer family members feel in the session, the more they will share things that are vulnerable, about which they are confused or stressed, about which they feel ashamed or guilty. Sharing these vulnerable things and the empathetic way in which they are handled by all involved in the session will contribute to the further development of safety in the session.

Simply inviting family members to speak freely in the session (which was called *free association* in traditional psychoanalysis) rarely leads to an unconcerned sharing of what is going on with the family members. The safety of speaking freely only succeeds as trust in the session grows.

---

Building a relationship of trust with each of the family members is a parallel and simultaneous process with building the working relationship: it also involves listening, empathy for suffering, and acknowledgement of commitment to a better life together. What is added specifically in relation to building trust is *respecting the way in which each of the family members tries to ensure their safety*: by keeping silent, by avoiding certain themes, by provoking conflicts in relatively safe areas, etc. This is often the key to building a good therapeutic relationship with family members who are hesitant to start therapy: he therapist does not know what the vulnerability is that is at stake, but he/she notices that the family member is trying to protect him/herself. In this way, the therapist shows that he/she senses that there is a vulnerability that needs protecting, and that he/she will try not to be a threat. The way in which someone protects him/herself is easier to see than the vulnerability that is protected. What is really vulnerable is safely hidden behind the protective wall. The wall can be seen, not what is behind the wall. The therapist sees how the family member is trying to protect him/herself and, and that offers the therapist a first clue about what the underlying sensitive strings that may be vibrating are. It is by giving the family member authentic recognition for the necessary protection, and appreciation for the family member who tries to take care of him/herself by protecting him/herself, that there may eventually be room for the family member to show what is so vulnerable that it needs this kind of protection. The sensitivity of the therapist gives the hesitant family member confidence, and so safety in the session can grow.

**Building a relationship of trust between family members**

The safety in the session depends not only on the therapist's relationship with the family members, but also on the relationship between the family members. This is related to the development of a working alliance in which the family members have a *shared sense of purpose*. They have roughly the same goal (to make family life better together), but it also means that the family members, despite the sometimes large differences that may exist in the family, and despite the different sensitive strings and the sometimes high-level conflicts, still feel a connection with each other. There must be a cohesion under the suffering and confusion; a bond that holds them together despite … I call that underlying bond *love*, but that bond can just as rightly be called a *loyalty bond* (Heyndrickx et al., 2022).

It may be difficult for the therapist to see the underlying bond between the family members. Family members typically begin therapy in emotional crisis, and they will mainly explain why they are worried, disappointed, or scared, and demonstrate this in the session. What the therapist gets to see in the beginning of the therapy are the conflicts, the mistrust, the fear, the anger, the despair, etc. The connection in the family (or the love that brought them together and perhaps still holds them together) seems absent. Love and connection at that moment are often no more than a vague memory of how it used to be in the family. However, the therapist has no choice: without connection or love in the family, family therapy makes no sense. Even if the therapist cannot perceive the implicit connection in the session, he/she must at least be able to *imagine* that connection. Otherwise, there is no hope for the family. In the midst of the overwhelming suffering in the family, the therapist can often catch a glimpse of connection and love here and there. This is expressed, for example, in the commitment that family members show – in fragments and moments – to make life better together. Those fragments and moments of connection are hopeful and important. The therapist must notice them, and at some point – at the *right* time – also name them; *without denying or minimizing the depth of suffering in the family.* Naming the connection must always go hand in hand with an empathy for suffering in the family, in the right balance and in the right order: first the empathy for suffering, and if the family members feel sufficiently recognized in their suffering, the connection in the family can also be mentioned. Often the first part of a first session is more focused on the individual family members and on the recognition of everyone's commitment and suffering, so that at the end of the session there may be some room to also mention something of the connection.

---

### You – You – ... – You-together-as-a-family

When the family therapist talks to a family, the conversation often has the basic structure of You- You - ... - You-together-as-a-family. First, the therapist listens to the story of the first family member and then gives a short empathetic paraphrase (You). Then the therapist invites the next family member to tell his/her story. The therapist listens and gives an empathetic paraphrase (You) after that story. This is how the family therapist listens to all the family members one-by-one. When every family member told his/her story about their worries, suffering, and commitment, the family therapist gives a new empathetic reflection, but this time addressed to the whole family (You-together-as-a-family).

So the therapist succinctly summarizes what each of the family members has said about their worries and their attempts to make it better (You-You-You- ...), and then focuses on the shared experience of the family (You-together-as-a-family).

Addressing the family as a whole can be done in different ways. For instance, the therapist can address them as a unit and focus on their shared suffering ("ou all feel exhausted"). The therapist may also talk about their shared experiences ("It must have come as a big surprise to all of you"), their shared struggle ("You are working hard to survive as a family") or about their common goal for therapy ("You come to therapy as a family, because you want to explore new ways to be together. Ways that are less stressful for all of you"). But it has to be done in the right balance and in the right order: always first acknowledging the different individual perspectives, before talking about the family as a whole.

## Maintenance of the alliance during therapy

Even after the first session, the therapist must deal with the therapeutic relationship with care. Throughout therapy, the alliance with each family member must be guarded, as well as the alliance with the family as a unit and their *shared sense of purpose*. Safety in the session is a concern throughout the therapy. When a family member's involvement appears low (e.g., the family member is remarkably silent or passive – as is illustrated in the case story of Lyka and her family, see chapter 8), this deserves the therapist's attention. The therapist must keep an extra eye on that family member and possibly address him/her to carefully explore what is going on. For example, the therapist may tell a hesitant family member that he/she has the impression that there is something that makes him/her quieter than usual: "I would very much like to understand it better; can you help me understand you better?" It is a delicate work, in which the therapist does not try to convince or persuade the family member. Psychoeducation and motivational techniques are out of place here. Usually, this is the best thing the therapist can do: listen to the family member in question and show genuine empathy for his/her feelings, experiences, and concerns.

Like in individual therapy, in family therapy too family members can become openly critical and angry, but they will rather withdraw from the conversation and remain silent when they are not happy with the way the therapy is going (Friedlander et al., 2019; Karam & Blow, 2023). Such silence of disappointment is usually not immediately noticed by the family therapist, whose attention may be occupied by another family member who is talking. Dealing with disappointment and with the impending early termination of therapy is more complex in family therapy than in individual therapy since everyone in the session may be involved in one way or another, and each has their own perspective. Metacommunication is necessary, but must be well guided by the therapist, who must also be present at the same time to listen to what is going on for the different family members.

---

**Feedback-orientation of the family therapist**

Systematically inviting family members to give feedback on how they experienced the session is helpful for the therapist to notice impending breakups more quickly. In chapter 7, feedback-oriented work is discussed in more detail.

---

Specifically for working with families, there is the additional risk of the *split alliance* (Glebova & Woolley, 2016; Escudero & Friedlander, 2017): the family therapist – sometimes seduced or pressured by some family members – identifies too strongly with certain family members at the expense of the others, who therefore feel that the family therapist is not on their side, or does not understand them sufficiently. A *split alliance* can weigh heavily on the family therapeutic process and often complicates a successful outcome of therapy (Friedlander et al., 2018).

---

**Research on split alliance and the outcome of family therapy**

In their meta-analysis on relationship and family therapy, Friedlander and her colleagues (2018) found, in addition to a strong link between the alliance and the outcome (effect size 0.62), an even stronger link between *split alliance* and *outcome* (effect size 0.66). This indicates that *split alliance* is often associated with a poor outcome of family therapy.

---

### The therapist and the therapeutic relationship

It requires a lot from the therapist to get a good therapeutic relationship with a family because the therapist must listen, understand, connect, ask questions, and intervene in a complex encounter in which the family members differ in experience, intention, fears, and wishes. The therapist must identify and differentiate with each of the family members; connect and disconnect. Each time the therapist breaks free from the empathic identification with the client, the therapist falls back on him/herself for a moment, only to begin the process again and reconnect with the next family member. Working with families is connecting with and empathizing with each of the family members, even though the different family members may have different concerns and different vulnerabilities, in a process of what Boszormenyi-Nagy called *multi-directional partiality* (Boszormenyi-Nagy & Sparks, 1973).

## Summarizing

We can depict some of the complexity of the therapeutic relationship in family therapy with three metaphors: the bridge, the wall, and the well.

1 Working on a good therapeutic relationship is about building a *bridge* (the connection between the therapist and the client; as well as between the family members themselves) where at first there was only emptiness, distance, and distrust.
2 It's also about respecting the *wall* (behind which the client can safely hide vulnerable things) and sensing what's precious and fragile behind that wall.
3 It's about creating safety for everyone so that they dare to explore the immeasurably deep *well* of their experiences, bringing out things from it that they want to share with others.

Building a good therapeutic relationship in family therapy is partly a matter of techniques (*what* should the therapist say to *whom* in *what way*) but – like an attachment relationship – it is mainly a matter of personal commitment and presence of the therapist. Byng-Hall (1995) emphasizes the importance of the therapist's *availability* to be a temporary attachment figure and a *secure base* for the family. Some talk about the importance of *being there* (Rober, 2008) or *presence* (Hayes & Vinca, 2017). Others talk about *responsiveness* (Watson & Wiseman, 2021): the therapist is present and gives an affirmative response to the input of each family member and invites each family member to express themselves further in the session. To live up to that responsiveness, the therapist must be close to the family members in the session: listening, empathizing, sensing, questioning, limiting, encouraging, protecting, challenging, etc. And yet the therapist must also keep his/her distance: keep an overview, form hypotheses, keep an eye on the time, evaluate whether the therapy is going well and adjust if things are not going well. It is a balancing act in which there is no specific balanced position. The therapist is flexible in movement and constantly changes position in response to what happens in the session, like a high-wire artist who keeps his/her balance on the rope by constantly making many small movements with his/her body.

# *Stairway to heaven*: Jason Sonck and his family (part 1)

"I don't want therapy. I want to d-d-d-die."

Jason's parents watched silently.

Mother used her handkerchief to dry her tears.

It was the first time I saw this family. It was immediately clear that something was wrong with Jason. My first thought was: this young man must have been in an accident or something that severely unbalanced his body and now it seemed to be feverishly searching to recover that balance. He was like a puppet on the strings of a clumsy puppeteer. It was strange to see such shocking helplessness in a beautiful, toughly dressed young man. Judging by his clothes, I couldn't help but think of a rock star.

I wouldn't hear Jason's story until later in the session, but I want to tell it now. He was a healthy young man until he had a motorcycle accident at the age of 22. A drunk driver drove him off the track. When the ambulance arrived at the scene of the accident, Jason was lying unconscious on the side of the road, bleeding from his nose and ears. He was taken to the hospital. The suspicion of a serious brain injury was confirmed in each new medical examination in the months that followed.

Jason was a guitar player with a fledgling rock band. Due to his brain injury, he had problems concentrating, memory problems, and splitting headaches. The band tried to make music together for a few more months, but Jason had changed. He could not concentrate for long, was easily irritated and short-tempered. If something didn't work out well, he could suddenly start cursing and throwing things. When he calmed down a little later, he retreated into a dark mood, unreachable to the others. After a few attempts to jam like in the old days before the accident, the band decided to take an indefinite break.

For Jason, this was terrible. Playing guitar was his life. He had put everything into becoming a good guitarist. Jimmy Page, Led Zeppelin's guitar wizard, had always been his hero. Page's guitar solo during *Stairway to Heaven* was the guitar nirvana for him. He practiced hard to play that

DOI: 10.4324/9781003458395-5

solo as well as he could, and he did a pretty good job. However, the accident had plunged him all the way down from his *Stairway to Heaven*. He no longer recognized himself in the broken guitarist he had become. He realized that he would never match Jimmy Page. In fact, he would even never match himself again. Never again would he become as good as he had ever been.

On the grounds of incurable and unbearable suffering, Jason requested euthanasia.[1] However, the doctor did not agree, and had said that it was impossible to predict what progress he could still make. He had referred him to the TBI (Traumatic Brain Injury) department of the teaching hospital. There, Jason repeated his request for euthanasia to the rehabilitation doctor in a conversation he had together with his parents. A discussion had ensued in which the parents encouraged Jason not to give up. That annoyed Jason. He became angry and reproached his parents for not understanding how difficult it was for him. The rehabilitation doctor suggested that they go into family therapy. The parents thought that was a good idea.

Now they were sitting here with me for the first family therapy session. They talked about Jason growing up: he was a sensible boy who did well in school and was loved by everyone. Music was Jason's great passion. Going to music school, listening to music with friends and discussing it. They then decided to form a band, and that band later gained its first fame through a final place in a well-known national contest for rock bands. Performances in small clubs followed, and later also some summer festivals.

It was quiet in the session. I had noticed that Jason had listened to what his parents were saying with a certain distance, without saying much himself: as if they were not talking about him, but about someone else.

I looked expectantly at Jason, for this silence gave him the opportunity to add or correct something, but he said nothing.

Father broke the silence: "Yes, now Jason lives with us again and now there are only concentration problems, headaches, memory problems, irritability, and so on."

He summed it up as if he were reading it off a paper.

It was quiet again.

Then Jason decided to speak anyway.

He said, "Yes, and n-n-n-now I want to d-d-d-d-die because life hurts and it makes no s-s-s-s-s-s-sense anym-m-m-m-more."

He said it too loudly, and then he was silent again.

Mother then said Jason's girlfriend had ended the relationship. It had been too hard for her: Jason with his mood swings and his anger attacks.

---

1 Euthanasia is legal in Belgium, even in some cases for non-terminal patients. Psychiatric patients can also request euthanasia when there is unbearable and hopeless suffering resulting from a serious and incurable disease or from an accident.

"We don't want Jason to give up," father said, "he has so many talents. And he can still play the guitar. Yesterday I heard him in his room."

"Phew. Yes, y-y-y-y-y-yesterday I messed around with my a-a-a-accoustic guitar. It was sh-sh-sh-shit."

Silence.

"How could family therapy help you?" I asked cautiously.

"I don't want f-f-f-f-f-fucking family therapy," Jason said. "I want to d-d-d-die."

"Mmm, ok," I said, "but we're sitting here together now, and we can talk together. How could this talk make sense to you?"

It was quiet for a moment.

"Maybe y-y-y-you can convince my parents to help me get eu-eu-eu-eu-euthanasia," Jason said.

Silence.

I turned to the parents: "And what do you hope to gain through family therapy?"

Mother looked at father.

He replied, "We want to help him come back alive. To really want to live again."

The sharp difference was immediately exposed on the table. I felt that this was going to be the challenge: How can I do therapy with this family, and sufficiently connect with each of these opposing questions? No, it would not be an easy therapy. That was immediately clear.

# Part II

# The family therapist in the session

# 3 The family therapist as a wounded healer

The importance of the person of the therapist was recognized early in the development of the field of family therapy. Bowen (1972), for example, emphasized that it is vital for therapists to break free from their own past and develop sufficient individuality within their own family-of-origin. Virginia Satir (2013, originally published in 1987) also wrote about the person of the therapist. She explains that the personality of the therapist together with the specific technique or therapeutic approach are crucial in the session. While the therapist's technique and person are sometimes seen in an either/or polarization, Satir suggests focusing on both. According to her, techniques and interventions are like tools: depending on who holds them, they are also used differently. In the past, the polarization between techniques and the therapist's person was more conspicuous in academic discussions, but nowadays – in line with Satir's ideas – there is recognition that the therapist brings theory and technique to the session and does so in a personal way. That is why it makes sense that a family therapy training – in addition to teaching protocols and interventions – also focuses on the person of the therapist, in order to optimize the therapist's ability to be aware of him/herself in the session and to use one's own person purposefully in the service of the development of the family (Aponte & Kissil, 2014).

## The therapist as a wounded healer

When the person of the therapist is discussed in a family therapy course, most approaches are based on the basic idea that a therapist is a *wounded healer* (e.g. Zerubavel, & Wright, 2012; Aponte & Kissil, 2014). With a historical lens, the therapist's past is explored and the focus is on meaningful events that have guided the therapist's development and that now may cause the therapist to stumble in his/her work with clients. It's a retrospective view.

DOI: 10.4324/9781003458395-7

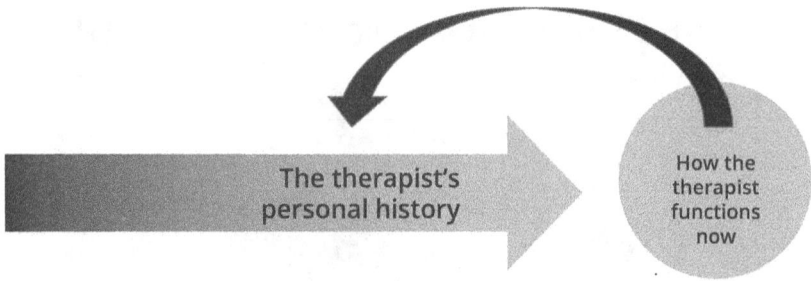

*Figure 3.1* A retrospective perspective.

Personal issues of the therapist can hinder the therapeutic work, and they can also have negative effects on the clients. The traditional psychodynamic view was that the therapist's problems had to be solved ("purification" - cfr. Freud, 1912, p. 116) in such a way that the therapist could be a blank screen for the client (Freud, 1912). Recent family therapeutic publications look at it differently: it is not about the therapist completely solving all his/her problems, but also about transforming someone's injury into an opportunity to be helpful or healing towards clients (Aponte & Kissil, 2014). Addressing the person of the therapist in training therefore actually serves a double function:

1 Protecting the client by solving the therapist's problems as much as possible. In this way, for example, the client can be protected against the narcissistic needs of the therapist, against his/her use of power, against the development of dependence (Satir, 2013), and so on.
2 Developing the competence of the therapist to use him/herself to help the client (e.g. Timm & Blow, 1999; Aponte & Kissil, 2014).

As mentioned earlier, the wounded healer work within a training program is *retrospective* and is usually framed as a form of family-of-origin work (e.g. Haber & Hawley, 2004). It is not only retrospective, but also *introspective* (Timm & Blow, 1999): the therapist is expected to become aware of his/her own history (experiences, traumas, deficits, assets, etc.) and is invited to reflect on ways in which these can play a role in his/her current professional functioning.

### The therapist's genogram

In most family therapy courses, training focuses on the trainees' family-of-origin by using genograms.

## Genogram

A genogram is a schematic diagram in which the composition of a family (in principle in at least three generations) is depicted. There are clear conventions about the symbols used for the family members: squares are men, circles are women, a crossed square or circle indicates that the person has died, etc.

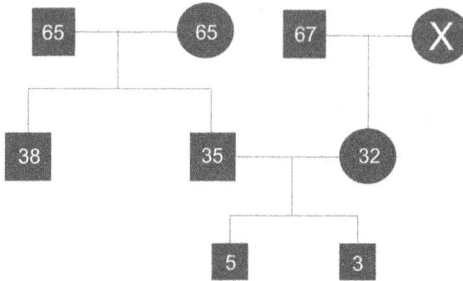

*Figure 3.2* A genogram.

Working with genograms in the field of family therapy goes back to a long tradition of intergenerational work in family therapy (Bowen, 1972; Boszormenyi-Nagy & Spark, 1973; Framo, 1992). The first publications on genograms appeared in the 70 s of the last century (e.g. Guerin & Pendergast, 1976). In contemporary family therapy, reference is still made to the impressive work on genograms by McGoldrick and Gerson (1985) which has had some adaptations and new editions over the years.

A family therapist in training is invited to explore his/her own developmental history, as well as his/her family history, and the question of what the trainee can learn from these reflections that could be useful for his/her functioning as a family therapist is posed. For example, the context in which the therapist grew up is considered: what were the challenges faced by the family (e.g. stress, illness, loss, trauma, etc.)? How were these challenges handled? What examples has the therapist had about being a man or being a woman? About how to love? On how to deal with problems? Furthermore, the position that the therapist took when growing up in the family-of-origin is also examined: Was he the scapegoat or the prince on the white horse? Was she the ugly duckling (who later turned out to be a swan) or was she the princess on the throne? It is often assumed that many therapists have previously had parentified roles in their family-of-origin (e.g. Jurkovic, 1997; Fussel & Bonney, 1990; Soloski, Turns, Schleiden, & Macey, 2016), and that they have already started to develop their skills as therapists there.

### Example genogram work with David:

David was a young therapist who followed our training as a family therapist. He was in the second year of the training, the year in which a significant part of the training time is spent on genogram work.

It had already been noticed in the supervisions and exercises that David could not handle conflicts well. He tried to avoid conflict as much as possible and when that didn't work, he was distraught and confused. Then he doubted himself as a therapist and during a certain supervision he wondered aloud whether he had the qualities to become a good therapist.

For example, there was that time when David wanted to talk with me as a supervisor about his therapy with the Rombouts family. The family consisted of a father and a mother with two sons, 16 and 18 years old, and the conflicts in the family sometimes ran high. They were conflicts between the sons and the parents, and sometimes between the sons themselves. It was remarkable that David felt responsible each time when another conflict between family members threatened to erupt in the session. He then began to work hard by leading the session, like a police officer controlling traffic. He asked one question and listened to the answer, anxiously trying to keep the others' reactions out of the conversation. Then he turned to another family member and talked to that family member while the others listened. He called on them to listen carefully to each other and not to interrupt when someone was speaking. That worked for a while, but it made him very central to the conversation, because there were no exchanges at all between family members without David's mediation. Then, at a certain moment, things went wrong and – despite David's attempts to contain everything – the conflict erupted in all its intensity. There was nothing to be done about it, but David felt defeated and exhausted. "I'm a failure," he told me. "Why the hell did I want to become a therapist?"

A few weeks later it was David's turn to present the genogram of his family-of-origin in the training group. David had made three geno-grams: one for the nuclear family (his parents who were divorced, his younger brother and David himself), one for his father's family-of-origin, and one for his mother's family-of-origin. I expressed my surprise at that:

"Most students have one genogram, and you have three," I said.

"My parents haven't talked to each other for 15 years. They split up when I was 14 and they both remarried. They live in very different worlds."

I went over the three genograms with David. It was remarkable how many cut-offs there were, not only between David's parents, but also within both their families-of-origin. The paternal grandmother had broken not only with her husband (divorce), but also with her own children. She didn't want to see them anymore and had started a new life with another man, with whom she had two more children. David's father's mother had left when she was 15. David's father did keep in touch with his father (Jan's grandfather), but he was angry with his father because, according to him, he was the cause of their mother abandoning them. There were also important cut-offs in the genogram of mother's family. In particular, mother had broken up with her brothers because of a legal issue concerning an inheritance after the death of their parents.

"There have been many conflicts in previous generations," David said, "I only noticed that when I was preparing for this genogram day. I wasn't really aware of it before."

"What were you most aware of?" I asked.

"Of the rupture between my parents, and of all the conflicts that preceded their separation," David said.

I asked David to explain this. He told the story of growing up in a family in which escalating conflict was imminent. He hasn't known it any other way. As a son, he noticed that he could sometimes do things to prevent conflicts from erupting in the family. The way that worked best was to talk to dad and try to understand him as best he could, and then talk to mom and try to understand her as best he could.

"Sometimes it worked," David said, "and that was a relief."

"So you've practiced how to deal with conflict in families from a young age?" I asked.

"Yes."

"And you've built up a lot of expertise in that area over the years? You learned very early on how to avoid conflicts at home?"

"Yes, but sometimes it didn't work. Then it went completely wrong. Then everything ended in a big great scolding, and I sat watching it. Paralyzed like a rabbit in headlights."

"And how did such a scolding stop?"

"Mother fled. She disappeared. Out of the house. We didn't know where she was. I was always relieved when she came back. My big fear was that one day she wouldn't come back."

"And that's exactly what happened to your father as a child? His mother didn't come back at some point?"

"Yes, I realize that now. I was apparently afraid that the same thing would happen to me, but I wasn't aware of that."

We talked for a while about David's family-of-origin. It became clear that it has been important for David all his life to avoid conflicts in his family because conflicts could lead to irreparable breakups. His family history was full of examples of such ruptures. It was also clear that David had learned a lot of interesting things in his role as a conflict avoider that could be particularly useful in his work as a therapist (e.g. securing by structuring, talking to each of those involved, empathetic listening, etc.). But his problem as a therapist was that he always used the same intervention method. In that way he wasn't flexible at all about dealing with conflict. While he mastered his intervention method very well and it often worked, he was still very vulnerable because when it didn't work, David was a mess, rather than an effective therapist.

"In addition to those assets you have, in what other ways could you, as a therapist, try to deal with difficult conflicts between family members in the session?" I asked.

David owed me the answer.

Other students in the group volunteered ideas:

"Let the conflict happen and thank them for demonstrating in the session how things are going at home," one student said.

"Ask parents what they learned in their family-of-origin about dealing with conflict," said another.

"Step outside the room, telling them that you'll come back when they've fought it out," said another.

There were several other ideas. Not all equally useful, but it was clear to David that there were still many things he could try out.

"Maybe you should try some of those things, David," I said, "That seems to me to be an important assignment for you during the training. Expand your arsenal. You have your assets, and you master them like a pro because you have practiced them many times. From an early age. But it would be good to become more flexible and add other useful stuff to your toolbox. And one very important thing you need to learn is that conflict doesn't necessarily lead to breakups. As a therapist, you have to accept that conflicts can arise in the session, and realize that you are not responsible for these conflicts."

### Therapeutic impasse

As illustrated in David's case above, family therapists in their clinical practices often stumble upon similar situations over and over again. This is called *therapeutic impasse* (Whitaker, Warkentin, & Johnson,1950): these are situations in which the therapist feels paralyzed and inadequate. It seems that he/she cannot do anything to restart the therapeutic process. That's what David experienced: impending conflicts in the session prompted him to use his expertise as a conflict avoider. However, when that didn't work, he was stuck.

An impasse means that the therapist is stuck on several levels (Flaskas, 2005):

1 *The therapist is narratively stuck*: what the therapist says about the family (to himself or to others) is poor, fixed, and rigid. The therapist's gaze is narrowed to a simplistic and one-sided vision.
2 *The therapist is psychologically stuck*: the attunement with the family and the curiosity of the therapist have disappeared, and instead the therapist clings to his/her vision of the matter and wants to see that vision confirmed by the family members.
3 *The therapist is stuck in his/her position vis-à-vis the family in the session*: the therapist is stuck in a position where he/she emotionally identifies too strongly with some family members in such a way that those family members feel understood by the therapist, and other family members feel misunderstood in the cold (*split alliance*).

### An example of an impasse:

A young family therapist called Jonas was working with family with a 17-year-old boy and his parents. Jonas was struck by the suffering and loneliness of the youngster and sympathized with him. From that position of identification with the boy Jonas tried to make the parents see that they should approach the youngster differently (e.g. have more understanding, lower expectations, be less restrictive, etc.). The result was that the parents did not feel seen in their commitment to their child, and that they felt that the therapist was on the side of their son. The more Jonas tried to convince the parents that they should approach their son differently, the more the parents felt neglected in their efforts to raise their son well.

In supervision Jonas talked about the therapy.

"I want to talk about this family because I think I'm stuck," Jonas told me.

His main feeling towards the family was frustration and irritation. He experienced the parents as stubborn and rigid.

I remarked that Jonas repeated each time that the parents should approach their son differently.

"You sound like an old record, repeating the same line every time,"

I said jokingly, "and also, you have lot of empathy for the boy – and that very good – but you seem to have no empathy for the desperation of the parents. On the contrary, you experience them as stubborn or rigid."

Jonas is a talented family therapist, and it didn't take long for him to see that he is fixed in a position close to the boy and far from the parents.

"I'm stuck in a split alliance," he concluded, and he was pleased with that conclusion as it gave him space again to reflect on his work with this family. His feelings of frustration and irritation had vanished. He said that he was eager to see the family again next week, and that he was going to start the session with apologizing to the parents for his stubbornness and rigidity.

## Flexible positioning and therapeutic alliance

The psychotherapy research I referred to in chapter 1 shows that the therapeutic relationship is very important for the effectiveness of therapy, and that the effective therapist is flexible and responsive towards the client. It also applies to family therapy, but, as I explained in chapter 2, in therapeutic work with *families*, the alliance is more complex than in individual therapy, and the flexibility of the therapist is even more important (Friedlander et al., 2018). It is this flexibility that is lost in the event of an impasse.

Instead of flexibility, there is a rigidity in positioning the therapist. That rigidity isn't really a motionless standstill like a statue; rather, it is a repetitive dance, with a repetition of the same simple dance steps with the family, and with accompanying repetitive thoughts of the therapist. The therapist's inner dialogue is poor and predictable: the same messages are repeated in silence. The messages are often also emotionally colored: the therapist is embarrassed, irritated, moved, angry, disappointed, afraid, desperate, etc. They are sometimes critical messages addressed to themselves: sometimes more humiliating or destructive ("You made a mess of it again, loser!"); sometimes more constructive and looking for a good approach ("I'm stuck, how do I get the process going again?"). They are also sometimes messages addressed to one or more family members (e.g. "Poor child, your parents don't understand you at all"). Sometimes it's an inner message of compassion or admiration ("Well said mother. Don't let that bully do that to you"). Sometimes the message is tinged with irritation and has reproachful or accusatory content ("If you would realize that you need to listen to her more, your daughter might not cut herself so much"). The therapist usually understands that he/she should not explicitly express such irritations in the session; they might be hurtful to some family members or antagonize them against the therapist. But what should the therapist do with what he/she cannot express in the session?

## Approaching the wounded healer through the impasse

One way to work with the wounded healer in training or supervision is to take the therapist's typical deadlocks – which he/she gets stuck in again and again – as a starting point. The well-known Italian family therapist Maurizio Andolfi, for example, started with his summer practicum in Rome in the late eighties, in which he worked with repeating impasses of the participants in what was called "handicap work". The basic idea was that every therapist has one (or more) handicap in addition to strengths and talents. These handicaps manifest themselves in his/her therapeutic work in a certain type of recurring impasse. Andolfi's training was aimed at transforming the handicap of a therapist into becoming "handi-capable" (Haber, 1990): by working in training with the therapist's impasses, the therapist can learn to see new possibilities and develop new skills.

In line with Andolfi's approach, Harry Aponte's *Person Of The Therapist* (POTT) training model focuses on *signature themes* (e.g. Aponte & Kissil, 2014; 2016). A *signature theme* is a psychological issue that is at the heart of the therapist's hurt, coloring his/her relationships with others (Aponte & Kissil, 2014). Aponte's focus is on the way signature themes are connected with themes in the therapist's life experience and family-of-origin. The goal of the POTT training is to address the *signature theme*, work through it as much as possible, and use it positively in therapy whenever it can support the therapeutic process: the more the professional is connected to his/her own life history and to his/her personal life now, the more he/she is available in contact with the family (Russon & Carneiro, 2016). In this way, the POTT training and supervision can help therapists to use their life experiences to better attune to their clients.

## Resonance as a sensitive string

In order to think about the therapist as a wounded healer, the concept of *resonance of the therapist* has been put forward in family therapy (Elkaim, 1997). The resonance of the therapist refers to the connection between the therapeutic process and the personal life of the therapist: in the session something happens that causes a sensitive string of the therapists to vibrate. When that happens, there are two interesting perspectives on the wounded healer in family therapy:

1 *The sensitive string*: What makes the therapist's string so sensitive? What can the sensitive string teach us about *the therapist and his/her history*?

2 *The vibration of the sensitive string*: How can we understand that the string is just now beginning to vibrate? What can we learn about *the family* from the vibration of the string?

## 1. The sensitive string

The first perspective on the wounded healer refers to the therapist's story and his/her history. It ties in with the perspective of the wounded healer.

### Example: Marianne and the vulnerable child

Marianne is a family therapist, and she has been coming into supervision for a while. During the supervision interviews, it becomes clear that Marianne repeatedly encounters families in which this pattern emerges: a hurt child faces parents who are disappointed and angry. Marianne always sides with the child. She can empathize with the loneliness and pain of the child, and she does not understand that the parents are impatient and disappointed in their child. Marianne then feels a powerless anger towards parents who seem unable to show sensitivity to their child. In that pattern, Marianne gets stuck over and over again.

The fact that Marianne repeatedly found herself in the same impasse was the signal for me to suggest to Marianne to reflect on her history, and in particular on her experiences in her family of origin. What is her story? How did she grow up? Who were her parents? Did she have siblings? What role did she have in the family? How did the family deal with setbacks, with pain, with loss, etc.?

### Example: Marianne and the vulnerable child (continued)

I was curious if the pattern of the hurt child versus the incomprehensible parents would recur somewhere in Marianne's history. I was well aware that as a supervisor I could not limit myself to looking for the repetition, because just noticing the repetition would only make Marianne more powerless, as her history would determine her to repeat the same pattern over and over again. I certainly didn't want to push Marianne into that powerless position. On the contrary, I wanted to help her feel like she had some *agency*. That's where I wanted to go with Marianne.

I realized that, in order to help Marianne to develop a sense of some *agency*, it was important to also look for the ways in which she had been struggling with the pattern of the hurt child and the parents who do not understand their child. I had to see what steps she had taken to deal with the difficulties. I also had to investigate where in her social network she had found support. I also wanted to know what partial solutions she had found, what hope there was in her history, and at what moments she had been free from the pressure of repetition: the so-called *unique outcomes* of Michael White (2007) or the *exceptions* of Steve de Shazer (1988).

Marianne told me that she had a brother who was two years older. However, he was mentally disabled and required a lot of care from the parents. As a result, they paid little attention to little Marianne, who was intelligent and socially skilled. And indeed, Marianne did very well in school and in the girl scouts. She was always a very independent child, and she could take care of herself.

"What my parents didn't see was that I was lonely and that I craved their attention and care," Marianne said. "But all the care from my parents went to my brother who really needed a lot of care. I understood that, but I still felt abandoned. They didn't see how I needed them. I've always stood by my parents and I've helped them where I could. Among other things, by not saying that I needed their attention and care, but in that silence, I was also angry with them because they did not see how vulnerable I was."

In Marianne's story we see the repetition. It is as if Marianne often finds herself in therapeutic work with families in situations like what she experienced in the past (her vulnerability that was not seen by her parents who were mainly focused on their mentally disabled son). They are often echoes of painful things from the past that were never articulated in the family.

"What helped you survive, and grow up to be a sensitive adult?" I asked Marianne.

Marianne was surprised by my question and was momentarily silent.

Then she replied: "I've learned to put up with a lot and go my own way quietly."

"That's nice. An important asset in life," I said, "and where did you find support?"

"My friends in the girl scouts. When I was with them, especially at the summer camps, I could forget my worries. Sometimes I could talk about things that hurt and that was good. Without my friends I might have survived, but it would have been so much harder and much less fun."

"I hear you've had a lot of good ideas for dealing with that difficult family situation: there were your talents, your intelligence, and your social skills. There was your love for your parents: you saw how difficult it was for them with your brother, and you wanted to avoid burdening them as much as possible. This is how you have learned to be strong and independent. You've also learned to seek connection outside of your family. You found that in your friends of the girl scouts ... If we put that together, those are impressive competencies that you developed there. How can these competencies help you as a therapist? What can you learn from this as a therapist?"

Again, Marianne was surprised by my question. She was silent for a long time.

"I don't know," she said, "can I think about that? I'll let you know what I think next time. Is that okay?"

Two weeks later we had the next supervision session. Marianne said she had talked to her parents a few days after the previous session.

"I just told them what I told you," she said, "and my parents were very happy that I told them. They were very moved, especially my dad. They said 'sorry'. Two days later I received a long letter from my father in the mail. Handwritten, you know, like the old days. In it, he thanked me for all I have done for them. I didn't expect that. I expected them to be hurt if I told them how it had been for me. Not that they would be grateful."

A few months later, at the end of her supervision process, I asked Marianne how she looked back at the evolution she had gone through as a therapist in recent months.

"The conversation with my parents was somehow a turning point. After that I felt freer to talk as a therapist about the different positions I saw in the family: the child who is vulnerable and does not feel seen, the parents who suffer from worries of all kinds and who rely on the child, the child who does not speak because he loves his parents and does not want to burden them ... I can look at what is happening in a family from those different positions, and I am no longer sucked into the position of the disgruntled and angry child as I used to be."

It is the hope of a supervisor that this kind of supervision work with a focus on the family of origin of the supervisee leads to a smoother and more effective functioning of the supervisee as a therapist. And often – as with Marianne – that also works. And when it works, a process of supervision is a bit like a therapeutic process through which things that were stuck become flowing again.

## 2. The vibration of the sensitive string

There is not only the question of what has made the wounded healer have a sensitive string. There is also a second perspective on the wounded healer and that is about the question: *what makes that sensitive string start to vibrate in this session?* What does it mean that the therapist gets stuck *with this family* and ends up in this rigid positioning? The therapist's "stuckness" doesn't only say something about the therapist and his/her history; it can also tell us something about the family.

The experience of the therapist can be seen as one of the aspects of his/ her listening (Rober, 2017b). After all, listening is not something you only do with your *ears*. You also do it with your *eyes* and that way you are responsive to the non-verbal aspects of the family members' story. But you can also do it with your *heart*: in the experience of the therapist, things are evoked that also tell a part of the story, especially that part that the client cannot capture in words and is also not able (yet) to express non-verbally. These are often the things that the client him/herself has little insight into; things the client cannot yet *mentalize* (Bateman & Fonagy, 2004). In the experience of the therapist, those non-mentalized things of the client are sometimes projected, as if the therapist were a white canvas on which a silent film is projected. If the therapist succeeds in bearing his/her experience (rather than immediately reacting), if he/she succeeds in getting those things sharp and in articulating them, then he/she can return those non-mentalized things of the client in the form of carefully formulated words and phrases. This can help the client to start to put his/her experience into words.

So there are opportunities here, but it is clear that this is also a difficult task for the therapist, who must move from his/her painful experience of being stuck in therapy in the direction of authentically dwelling on the vibrating of his/her sensitive string and then go even further and investigate what may have been expressed by the client in the vibrating of the string. How does the therapist's string vibrate with a string of one of the family members? This is a difficult question for the therapist alone, and in this the help of a supervisor can often be very useful.

This second perspective on the wounded healer is fascinating and complex. It deserves a more detailed discussion. Such discussion can be found in chapter 6 of this book when we talk about the therapist's self-supervision and the therapist's reflection in his/her inner dialogue.

## Conclusion

The retrospective work around the person of the therapist in training and supervision is not tied to one therapy model. It transcends models and could well be seen as an approach that responds to common therapy factors (Morgan & Sprenkle, 2007; Karam & Blow, 2023). Either way, this kind of work should have a place in any family therapy training, regardless of the model or protocol one wants to promote (Scott & Wendt,

2018). After all, training and supervision of family therapists should be aimed, in addition to teaching models and protocols, to help them develop their ability to form good therapeutic relationships in their work with families. While this is likely to involve learning certain skills and techniques, it is also necessary to pay attention to the therapist's personal history (e.g., Aponte & Carlsen, 2009; Regas, Kostick, Bakaly, & Doonan, 2017). One might even consider putting this kind of work around the therapist's person at the center of family therapy training (Simon, 2006).

# 4   The family therapist in action

In addition to the historical/retrospective perspective on the person of the therapist that I discussed in the previous chapter, there is another perspective that is important when we consider the family therapist in the session: the *present moment* or *in-the-process* perspective. The focus is not on the personal history of the therapist, but on the person of the therapist in the present moment of the session.

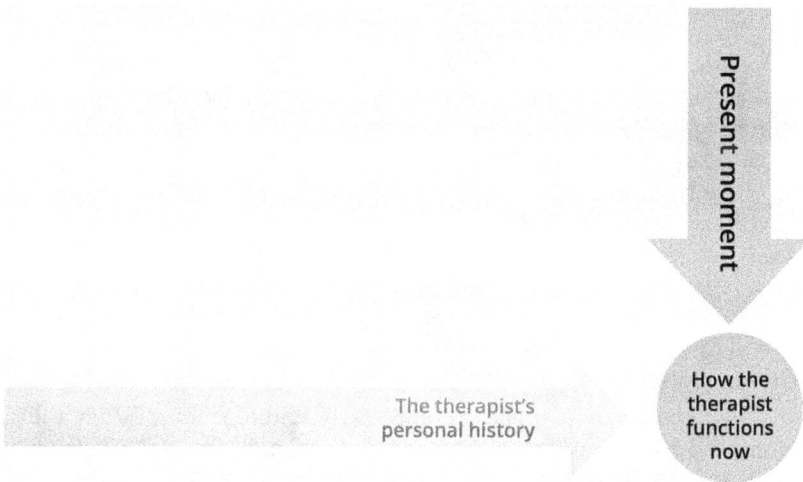

*Figure 4.1* A present moment perspective.

In order to illustrate what I mean exactly with this perspective I want to tell a case story.

## The story of Sofie and her family

Sofie and her family were referred by the family doctor. Five months ago, Sofie (five years old) had been sexually abused by her uncle Jos

DOI: 10.4324/9781003458395-8

(mother's younger brother). We (my young colleague Alien Hoorelbeke and myself) invited the family for a first session.

That morning, Alien and I were preparing the session in my office. We didn't have much information beforehand, but we realized it was a delicate situation with a very young girl being abused by someone in the family. Then I realized that I had forgotten to ask the family's permission to video-tape the session. As I knew the family was already waiting in the waiting room, I said to Alien, "Wait here, I will go to the waiting room and ask for permission."

Our waiting room is a big room with about a dozen chairs and when I entered, I saw the family sitting on the other side of the room: father, mother, Sofie and Sofie's brother Ronny (eight years old). My intention was to head for the parents and ask their permission to videotape the session, but at that moment I saw Sofie. She was feeding a baby doll with a toy bottle. I made eye contact with Sofie and with some hesitation I went straight to Sofie.

I got down on my knees and I asked her the name of her baby. Sofie did not stop feeding the doll when she said: "She's called Rosalie."

I said: "Hi, Rosalie," and touched the baby on the cheek. "Nice to see you have a mother who takes good care of you."

I made eye contact with Sofie when I said the word "mother". Sofie beamed and glanced at her mother who gave her a big smile in return. I addressed Sofie and said: "Let me introduce myself, I'm Peter."

"I'm Sofie," she said.

"Nice to meet you," I said, and I addressed the boy sitting next to her: "And you must be Ronny. Nice to meet you." I shook his hand. Then I moved to the left and said hello to the mother and the father. I shook their hands. Then I asked them permission to video-tape the session. The parents said "Of course," and checked with both children. For them it was ok too. I said: "Thanks. We'll begin in a few minutes."

When I entered my office, I immediately said to Alien, "What a nice family!" I added: "When we go and meet them in the waiting room, I think it is important for you to say hello to Sofie first." I explained what had happened in the waiting room and I said, "I think it is best to also get down on your knees and greet the baby first, and then Sofie."

Alien was surprised and asked: "Euh, ok, but why?"

I replied: "I don't know why. It feels right, that's all. First say hello to Sofie and her baby –she's called Rosalie. And then to Ronny and then to the parents." Alien didn't understand why I advised her to meet the family like this, and neither did I.

She insisted: "On my knees? Why?"

I had no immediate answer. I reflected for a moment and I tried to explain: "When I went to the waiting room, I wondered how to make contact with Sofie and I understood that it would not be easy. Then I saw them sitting there, and I noticed that Sofie was feeding her doll. I went to Sofie and I greeted the doll first. I addressed Sofie as a good mother. In that way I made contact with the three of them; the doll, Sofie, and her mother. I connected with them and that felt right." This explanation may make sense in retrospect, but it was not what had steered my actions in the waiting room. My actions didn't originate from any explicit reasoning, but rather seemed to emerge in the moment. They felt to be automatic and as I was in the process, I acted in response to what happened between Sofie, her family, and me.

A few minutes later, when we met the family in the waiting room, Alien did just as I had proposed, and I could see that she immediately had a good connection with the children. Then she went to the parents shook their hands. We went to the consultation room.

The children entered the room first, chose a seat, and sat down. Then father sat down and finally mother entered. When she sat down in her seat, she gave a big sigh. It sounded like a sigh of relief. I addressed her and said, a bit jokingly: "What a big sigh. What's the story of that sigh?"

Mother said: "I feel we are in the right place."

"In the right place? What do you mean?"

Then mother said: "The last time the four of us were sitting in a waiting room was in the police station. We had to go there to talk about what happened to Sofie, and it was so different from the way you handled it here."

Then mother told the story of them sitting in the waiting room at the police station, scared and confused by what had happened. A female police officer came out of one of the offices and came to pick up Sofie for her interview. "Give your doll to your mother, and come with me," the officer said. Sofie reacted confused and turned to her mother for help. Mother tried to reassure her and said: "I will go with you." But the officer was strict: "No, you stay here. I want to talk to your daughter alone." The officer took Sofie to her office for the interview. When Sofie sat in the chair in front of the big desk, the officer asked her: "Tell me, what has happened?" Sofie didn't dare to speak. The officer asked: "Your uncle, what did he do to you?" Sofie kept silent. When the officer became irritated Sofie closed off even more. Whatever the officer tried, Sofie did not say a word. After a few minutes that officer took Sofie back to the waiting room.

"You see," mother said to me, "when I saw you entering the waiting room, I was scared that something like that would happen again here, but it didn't. You went to Sofie. You went down on your knees and talked to her. You said hello to Rosalie. You told Sofie she took good care of her baby. You were respectful. And then when we entered this room, we immediately saw the toys and we knew that children are welcome here. Yes, that was a relief."

The story of Sofie and her family is an illustration of the challenge of meeting a new family and starting to form a therapeutic alliance. It illustrates that a good alliance builds on simple and humane connections. Furthermore, it illustrates that the start of a therapeutic alliance is sometimes tainted by previous alliances with helpers that have gone wrong. It is clear that our meeting the family had become more difficult by what happened in the police station.

Besides the challenge of forming a therapeutic alliance, there is another interesting aspect of this story. When I went to the waiting room it was my intention to ask for permission to video-tape the session. However, rather than addressing the parents, I went to the girl, got on my knees and talked with her about Rosalie, her doll. What happened there has made me think about being a family therapist in the living process of actual therapy. We can learn protocols about how to do therapy, we can have plans and good intentions. But what do we actually do in response to our clients in the present moment? It seems we don't always know what we do, nor why. Yes, we can come up with an explanation afterwards, but does that explanation offer us the real reason why we did it? It is also interesting in this case that we have the mother's feedback (her sigh of relief and the story about the police interview) that at least suggests that what we did – without planning it and without actually knowing why we did it – made sense in the context of our meeting with Sofie and her family.

The meeting with Sofie and her family in the waiting room will be the case in point in this chapter and my main question will be: *how can we understand what happened to me at that moment?* I want to focus specifically on my straying from my original intention to ask permission to video-tape the session, and on what I did seemingly automatically – without much reflection. In fact, in retrospect I can see that I did things that I would never recommend to my students (as an adult male therapist, immediately moving so close to a young girl whom you never met before and whom you know has been sexually abused by a grown man). Still the feedback of the mother (and at the end of the session also the feedback from another family member, obtained using a client feedback question-naire) confirmed that my move had been appreciated by them.

## The therapist's experiences in the process

In the present moment perspective, the focus is on what the therapist actually does in the session with the family as well as on the therapist's self-reflection (e.g. Flaskas, 2012) and on the whole range of experiences the therapist has in the session (e.g. Rober, 2011). This perspective is central for instance in the supervision approach that is focused on the therapist's inner dialogue (e.g. Rober, 2017a), in which the focus is on the dialogue between the therapist's experiencing self and his/her professional self (Rober, 2005b), as well as on the creation of reflective space (Flaskas, 2002; 2012).

Several authors have emphasized that the personal experiences of a therapist can be a source for creative interventions (e.g. Andolfi, Angelo, & de Nichilo, 1989; Whitaker & Keith, 1981; Wilson, 2007). The sharing with the client of the therapist's own associations, fantasies, and bodily sensations is not uncommon for these therapists. Furthermore, according to some authors what the therapist experiences during the session is particularly meaningful as it sometimes tells part of the client's story (Rober, 2017b): our clients make us feel what it is like to live their lives (e.g. Flaskas, 2002). What the client is not able to express in a verbal or a non-verbal way is sometimes reflected in what the therapist experiences. We have to listen to our own experiencing process in order to better understand the stories of the family members (Rober, 2017b).

---

**Intersubjectivity and the present moment**

In his book *The Present Moment*, Daniel Stern (2004) discusses the therapeutic relationship in terms of intersubjectivity. It is no longer about the two subjects (therapist and client) but a kind of third pole arises that can be called intersubjectivity. It is about interacting with the other with an unspoken understanding that "I know that you know that I know" and "I feel that you feel that I feel". Stern draws our attention to the fact that in our contacts with others we try to anticipate their behavior and we can respond to a certain extent to the feelings, thoughts, and intentions of the other, without these being made explicit by him/her (neurologically speaking via our mirror neurons). In doing so, we base ourselves on subtle and fine nonverbal signals (facial expression, posture, movement, voice, etc.): "a sort of direct feeling route into the other person is potentially open and we resonate with and participate in their experiences, and they in ours" (Stern, 2004, p.

76). The word "potentially" is interesting in this quote. It points out that this emotional resonance is not always present: sometimes we resonate well with someone, and sometimes we don't. We can then start thinking about the conditions for such moments of resonance: what is needed for two subjects to succeed in developing a rich intersubjectivity?

Stern first carefully studied the interplay between two people in mother-baby interactions. He has written beautiful books about this (e.g. Stern, 1985). Later he extended his ideas to other relationships (therapeutic relationship, romantic relationship, etc.) (see e.g. Stern, 2004).

Intersubjectivity is a dealing with each other from an implicit understanding of each other's inner world. Implicit then means; *I behave smoothly and fluently as if I know or feel what is going on with you, but if you ask me to explicitly explain what is going on with you, then that is not easy and then I hesitate and feel that I need time to think about it.* Intersubjectivity can be described as the mental landscape in which you and I move; it arises naturally from our dealings with each other when we have contact.

Daniel Stern shows how our nervous system is set up to allow us as human beings to transcend our subjectivity, to resonate emotionally and cognitively with someone else, and to create intersubjective moments. These are moments that we mutually share and in which we participate in another's lived story. It is interesting to note that we can do that without losing our subjectivity. After all, this is not about fusing with someone. No, *I* remain *me*, and *you* remain *you*, but – by empathizing with each other and feeling good about each other – a third pole is created (1 + 1 = 3). That third pole is a mental landscape in which we share things with each other, and in which we also shape each other's inner lives (feelings, thoughts, intentions, etc.). "In short, our mental life is cocreated", Stern writes (2004, p. 77).

Being sensitive to one's own experiencing is no simple matter. Most authors agree that the therapist has to be aware of his/her own experiences; to bear them, to tolerate them, and to reflect on ways to use such experiences in the session (e.g. Flaskas, 2005). I myself have written for instance, that a family therapist needs to take time for this process, instead of acting impulsively on his/her emotion, without any reflection (Rober, 2011). While this makes sense, acting without reflection was exactly what I had done in the waiting room with Sofie. I automatically followed my impulse to meet with Sofie first, instead of asking the parents for permission to videotape the session as had been my well-reflected intention. I acted in the moment, as if I knew what I was doing, but I didn't. I did it intuitively.

## The therapist acting intuitively

What is *intuition* exactly? The concept has been an important object of study and reflection in a wide range of cultural fields: philosophy, psychology, religion, spirituality, parapsychology, the arts, and so on. The meaning of the concept might also be different depending on the field in which it functions. Furthermore, it is a concept that is often treated with suspicion in the academic world, especially with regard to clinical judgment in medicine and clinical psychology (e.g. Dawes, 1994). Research in cognitive psychology has warned us of the deceptive nature of intuitive judgment of professionals. Meehl (1954) for instance showed how intuitive clinical predictions are far less accurate than statistical algorithms. Meehl's publication was the starting point of a deep controversy in the field of clinical psychology, and lead to a tsunami of studies comparing clinical predictions with statistical ones. All these studies pointed in the same direction: statistical prediction is at least equally effective or superior to clinical prediction (Kahneman, 2011).

The cognitive psychological research on clinical predictions may however not be so relevant for clinical practice, as making predictions is only a small portion of clinical judgment and of a clinician's expertise (Westen & Weinberger, 2005). Furthermore, Klein & Hoffman (2008) have emphasized that a lot of the findings of cognitive psychological studies on decision making stem from artificial laboratory research and that decision making in the real world is different. Therefore, researchers have focused their efforts on studying naturalistic decision making (e.g. Klein, 2015). The decision making of professionals from diverse fields has been investigated: firefighters, police officers, doctors, chess players, and so on. In all of these domains it seems that automatic cognitive processes are important, besides more deliberate ones. Engel (2008) for instance studied medical expertise and he made the distinction between implicit and explicit reasoning. Explicit reasoning is analytic, deliberate, and slow. Implicit reasoning is automatic, fast, and intuitive. It is a kind of embodied expertise that has been described before: Schön (1983) has called it *knowledge-in-action*, and – even earlier – Polanyi (1958) used the term *tacit knowledge*.

## Implicit knowledge

In his book *The Present Moment*, Daniel Stern (2004) discusses the importance of knowledge that is implicit in our actions. What we actually do and the knowledge that is present in our actions cannot be disentangled. This is different with explicit knowledge: explicit knowledge is somewhat separate from our actions (it is a kind of *pausing* that we are doing in order to think). Furthermore, explicit knowledge is symbolic and verbal knowledge. It is a kind of knowledge in which something is claimed about that world, and which assumes a certain distance from the world.

Stern states that a child is only able to use explicit knowledge when he/she has learned to master the language (+/- 18 months). All interactions of the baby with his/her environment before (approximately) 18 months exclusively lead to implicit knowledge. It is knowledge that directs the baby's actions but is not verbalizable or symbolic. It is about self-knowledge (implicitly having a sense of one's own experiences); knowledge about others (implicitly having a sense of what others experience); and knowledge about the world (implicitly having a sense of what is happening in the environment). It is a knowledge that is intertwined with action, and where there is no mediation of language or reflection. Bowlby's working models of attachment are an example of such implicit knowledge, in which the child's experience of what is safe and what is not, and how best to deal with insecurity, is condensed (Bowlby, 1969).

In older children and adults, both implicit and explicit knowledge are present. They are intensely intertwined in our lives, but they remain to a large extent separate domains. With some effort, implicit knowledge can sometimes also be made explicit by dwelling on it, naming it, and reflecting on it. It is possible to reflect on myself (*how do I feel? What do I want?*); on others (*how does my mother feel? What does my father expect from me?*); and on the world (*Is it going to rain today? What is the best strategy to solve this mathematical problem? What is the fastest route to my holiday destination?*). But not all our implicit knowledge is made explicit. For example, our language skills are largely based on implicit knowledge: I know how to speak my native language (Flemish/Dutch), but speaking, understanding, and writing happens automatically without explicit awareness of the language rules at play in my native language. I follow the rules but I don't have to make them explicit in order to do so. In fact, this is how it

> goes with most implicit knowledge that governs our dealing with ourselves, with each other and with the world: we use that knowledge in our daily actions without being aware of it.

The distinction Engel (2008) makes between explicit and implicit reasoning is similar to the distinctions made in cognitive psychological dual process theories of higher cognition (social cognition, judgment, decision making, reasoning, etc.) (e.g. Stanovic & West, 2000; Evans, 2003, 2008). The exact terms used by these theorists differ (Evans, 2008): implicit vs. explicit, intuitive vs. reflective, non-analytic vs. analytic, automatic vs deliberate, fast vs slow ... Still, all these terms seem to refer to a similar duality in our cognitive functioning: our behaviour is governed by two parallel cognitive processes that work together (Evans, 2008); with one more dominant part of the time, and the other more dominant the rest of the time. The distinction between these two cognitive processes is often regarded as one of the most important distinctions in cognitive science (Sun, 2015).

The best-known cognitive dual process model is that of Nobel Prize winner and psychologist Daniel Kahneman (2011). He makes a distinction between *system 1* and *system 2*:

- *System 1* is automatic, holistic, and has a high capacity. There is no sense of voluntary control but rather one of some kind of alienation: *I act and I can observe myself doing it but it somehow feels like it happens to me*. This cognitive system uses intuitive, bodily knowledge to act in tune with the context in which one functions. This knowledge has been built up through living our lives and developing patterns that enable us to rapidly size up situations and make immediate and implicit decisions, without losing time and without explicitly considering different options. This process can be referred to as "fast thinking" (Kahneman, 2011).
- *System 2* is deliberate and takes mental effort. It proceeds sequentially, step-by-step: *I consciously reflect in an explicit and more or less orderly way*. This cognitive system is of critical importance as *system 1* is not always reliable. Sometimes *system 1* may orient us towards our goals, but at other times it leads us astray. Luckily, we have a *system 2* that monitors what we are doing in the moment. *System 2* watches, evaluates, considers, and re-considers. It is like a "comparator" (Gray, 2007), as it compares one's expectations with what actually happens. Maybe it is also like an "interpreter" (Gazzaniga, 2013): it interpets the bits and pieces of information and tries to make

coherent sense of it all. It makes us aware of some of the cognitive processes that were implicit only moments ago. But *system 2* also takes time as it is hard to become aware of intentions and plans (e.g. Libet, Gleason, Wright, & Pearl, 1985). Experiments in cognitive psychology suggest that our awareness is always just after the fact (about 300ms); never in the present moment (e.g. Posner & Snyder, 2004). *System 2* can be referred to as "slow thinking" (Kahneman, 2011).

---

### The embodied mind

In contemporary psychology, the Cartesian distinction between body and mind is fundamentally questioned. In the past, it was assumed that one thinks and makes plans first, and that then one executes those plans by acting. That idea is now outdated. In its place comes the idea of the *embodied mind* (Varela, Rosch, & Thompson, 1992). The basic idea is that our thinking does not precede action, but that our thinking is largely *in* our actions.

For example, there is a whole series of cognitive psychological theories that state that our thinking and acting are cognitively based on the unconscious anticipation of events. According to Clark (2019), for instance, we are enmeshed in circular causal flows that intimately bind acting and perceiving: without thinking about it, we constantly make predictions in our actions based on our experiences, and our actions are guided by whether or not our predictions come true. We are not focused on perceiving the world and thinking about the world; we are focused on being part of the world, interacting with it. In that interaction, it is not possible to tell perception, cognition, emotion, and behavior apart. Body and mind form one integrated whole in interaction with the environment. If we have time to pause and think about it, then we can retrospectively analyze our actions, what we observed, what we experienced, what we thought, etc. But such reflections on our behavior are slow and they assume distance and time. It's something we can only do in retrospect.

---

According to Kahneman (2011), *system 1* and *system 2* are both continually active while we find our way through our world. Most of the time, *system 1* is on the foreground, and *system 2* is in stand-by mode.

When all goes well *system 2* doesn't interfere with *system 1*'s automatically steering our behaviour. But now and then, especially when *system 1* is confronted with something surprising, puzzling, or out of the ordinary, *system 2* – the comparator (Gray, 2007) – becomes more active in order to reflect on the issues at stake. Attention is focused now. More detailed and explicit considerations are made. Different options are weighed, and that takes time. A course of action is planned and performed. *System 2* monitors the intended steps and evaluates the outcome. When things run smooth again, *system 2* eases down and returns to its stand-by mode. In that way the intuitive *system 1* is balanced by the deliberate and analytic *system 2*.

### The Story of Sofie and her family (continued)

It is not so difficult to use the dual process frame to make sense of what happened in the waiting room when I met Sofie and her family. When I entered the waiting room with the intention of asking permission to make a video recording (a plan made up by *system 2*), I saw Sofie. Immediately I acted without thinking, abandoning my initial intention and letting myself go in the process of responsive attunement (Rober, 2017b) with the girl and, as it happens, with the whole family.

In retrospect, what I did was strange and puzzling: I don't usually get on my knees when I meet families for the first time in the waiting room. With Sofie's family I did. It somehow happened and while it was happening it felt natural and harmonious. During the whole sequence I had eye contact with Sofie, while she kept an eye on me. I sensed that what I did was in tune with Sofie. Every next move I made was welcomed by her. Also, the other family members seemed to appreciate my words and actions. And that encouraged me to make the next move. In retrospect I can see that I proceeded step by step, not guided by some kind of preconceived mental plan or protocol, but rather by the immediate responses my steps evoked in the others. I was responsive to the family and in some way a pleasant atmosphere was emerging between the family members and me as we gradually became more attuned to one another.

While Kahneman's *system 2* was standing by, the intuitive *system 1* was leading the way. However, in retrospect I realize that my actions didn't just emerge in the moment but that they were also connected to things I have learned in the past. The teachers who inspired me most as a young therapist (Edith Tilmans-Ostyn, Salvador Minuchin, Maurizio Andolfi, etc.) have taught me to focus on children when working with families. Andolfi, for instance, wrote that the child can be addressed as a consultant, who – as the thread of Ariadne – can lead the therapist through the labyrinth of a family session (Andolfi, Angelo, & de Nichilo, 1989; Andolfi, 1995). I learned a lot from these ideas of Andolfi: when I meet families for the first time in the waiting room I tend to focus on (often modestly) connecting with the children in the family. I have special attention for them, and I am oriented toward opportunities to make contact. I learned that often there are subtle invitations of some kind: things they say, or the message on their T-shirt, or toys they bring ... I look for an appropriate way to connect with the children, and sometimes succeed in making an explicit and overt connection in the waiting room. With some children, however, the appropriate way to meet them is limited to discrete eye contact or a formal handshake. I have learned that it is a process of *responsive attunement* (Rober, 2017b). My openness to what Sofie was doing in the waiting room did not mysteriously emerge from some deep well of mystical intuition. It is more like the final stage of a learning process: when I started out as a young family therapist, I had to proceed cautiously when I met a family and it needed all my attention. But after practicing family therapy for 30 years it seems that I have succeeded in translating my practical experience as a family therapist into intuitive action that feels automatic and that I can reflect on retrospectively.

So when I entered the waiting room my focus on meeting the children must have kicked in. A few minutes later, when I went to my office to pick up my colleague Alien, I regained some mental space to reflect on what had happened (*system 2* became more dominant). With her questions Alien helped me to reflect on my actions. I remember I welcomed her questions because they made me think, but I also felt that my words failed to convincingly explain to her (as well as to myself) what had happened.

### The person of the therapist in the process

If we use the frame of the models of cognitive psychologists like Kahneman and others, we can say that what cognitively drives the therapist in the family therapy process is a dual process, in which there is a dynamic tension between the two complementary cognitive systems:

- *System 1* or *fast thinking:* without much explicit reflection the therapist intuitively acts in the flow of the dialogue, responsively immersed in a shared *we* with the family. The therapist is sensitive to what happens in the session, groping for a good attunement with the client. The presence of the therapist (Hayes & Vinca, 2017) and immediacy (Hill et al., 2019) are central here. This is *the responsive therapist*; the therapist as part of the intersubjectivity with the family (Stern, 2004).

- *System 2* or *slow thinking*: the therapist has a plan and observes what happens, evaluates his/her own actions in the session, thinks of new ways to approach certain themes, and so on. The therapist is a spectator of what happens in the session, including his/her own actions. This is the therapist as a *self-supervisor*, who as an *I* oberves the actions of the *we* of which he/she is part, and who reflects on this *we*.

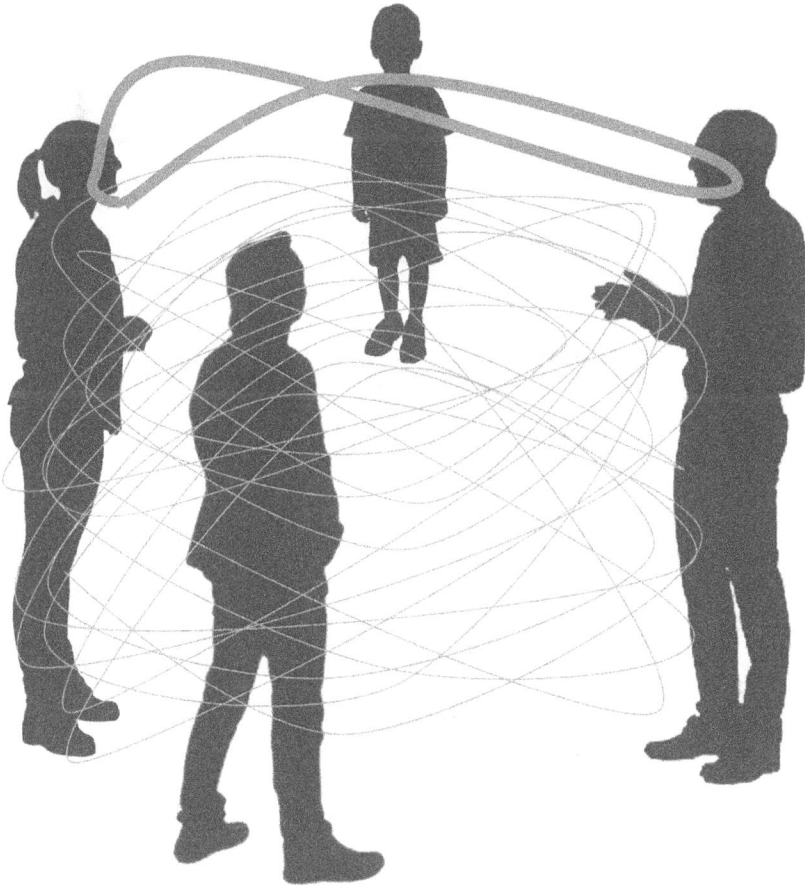

*Figure 4.2* System 1: Intuitive, responsive.

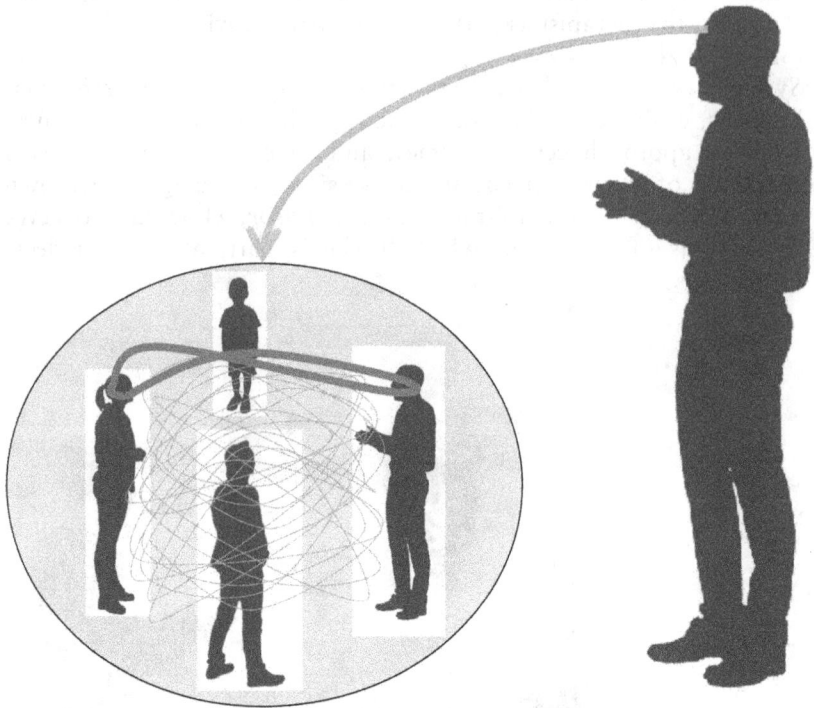

*Figure 4.3* System 2: Reflection, self-supervision.

It is important to keep the distinction between *system 1* and *system 2* in focus. We are most familiar with thinking from *system 2*, because this is the functioning as described by traditional psychology: a person has a goal, makes a plan to achieve the goal, executes the plan, and finally evaluates whether the goal has been achieved.

> For example: a man is hungry, decides to go to the bakery to buy a croissant. He does so and afterwards he finds that his hunger has been satisfied. Goal achieved.

According to the traditional psychological view, the person is goal-oriented and self-aware. The person acts in a world of people and things that are delineated from each other and can be named. Things have characteristics that we can get to know. We recognize causal relationships in their interactions: one thing is the cause and the other is the effect. That's the world of billiard balls, Bateson (1979) would say. It is the world that we can look at from the outside, and that the therapist gets to know through his/her observations. The therapist is mentally separate from the world in which he/she moves and that gives room for reflection.

But a therapist is not an observer all the time. He/she is also absorbed in the interaction with the family in the session and at those moments *system 1* dominates the cognitive functioning of the therapist. A therapist who acts intuitively and responsively in the session is, as it were, part of an eco-system that is fluidly in the making in the moment. It is a continuous flow of events that does not come to an end point but stretches out ever further in the future. And most things in the flow are not clearly delineated from each other, as everything is connected. Things are difficult to name, and words fail because things in this world often escape the words we are trying to capture them with. There is often no cause and effect that can be clearly distinguished because what is there usually has a complex history in which causes usually lead to all kinds of consequences, which in turn cause different things. The therapist himself/herself is also indistinguishable as a person in the intersubjectivity that he/she forms together with the family members.

> For example, the therapist sometimes senses what family members are going through and if he/she is responsive the family members feel understood in something that in their opinion they have not expressed, and that can surprise them because sometimes the therapist seems to understand them better than they understand themselves.

Also, our communication often runs smoothly as the answer is already given before the question is fully pronounced. In that flow of interactions, the therapist is immersed together with the family members. Yes, to describe the therapist functioning in *system 1*, our language becomes blurrier and more fluent, because in this world the therapist is not remote as an observer, but he/she is a part of the intersubjectivity that is always in motion and is never finalized. The therapist is with the family members, and functions intuitively, without much reflection in response to the context in which he/she moves.

The flow of the living world in which the therapist is immersed when he/she functions in *system 1* never stops and everything happens for yet another first time (Shotter, 2016). The therapist can at times withdraw from that world and distance him/herself. This way he/she can observe the world from a mental distance and name things. Then the therapist's functioning is governed by his cognitive *system 2* and he/she can name his/ her own experiences, set goals, make plans, etc., to then immerse themselves in the world again and be part of it.

We could illustrate this schematically in this way:

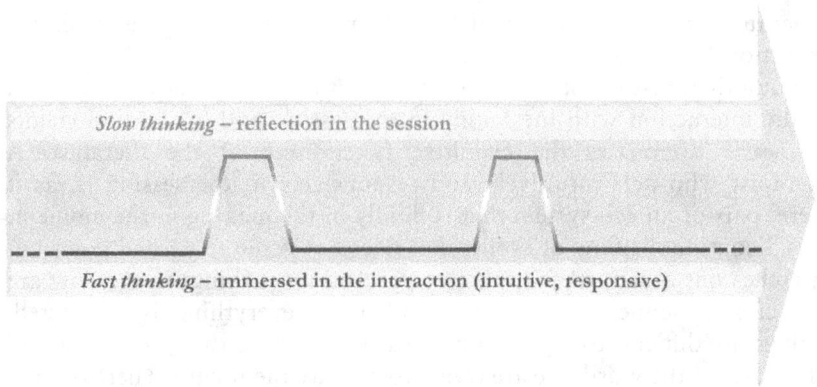

*Slow thinking* – reflection in the session

*Fast thinking* – immersed in the interaction (intuitive, responsive)

*Figure 4.4* The therapist in action: the oscillation between two cognitive systems.

Viewed in this way, the therapist's actions are intuitively responsive and bodily in the first place (*system 1*): as therapists we are oriented towards the family members and immediately our body has a response ready, and then, a few milliseconds later (Posner & Snyder, 2004), as if it were an epiphenomenon, there is our awareness of our choices: our explanations, our reflections, our hypotheses, etc. These more explicit cognitive activities originating from *system 2* are in constant dynamic tension with our more tacit, bodily responses from *system 1*; monitoring them, reinforcing them, correcting them, inhibiting them, etc. I am my own supervisor.

### Two *homunculi?*

Actually, our cognitive functioning as therapists probably isn't as simple as it is depicted here. I describe the process as if the therapist is in fact two *homunculi*: on the one hand an intuitive, responsive therapist, and on the other hand a self-supervisor who has more mental distance and reflective space, and who keeps a close watch in order to intervene when necessary.

---

#### *Homunculus*

*Homunculus* is Latin for *little man*. In psychology, consciousness is sometimes personified, as if there is a little person in the person who perceives things, who thinks, and who then makes decisions. This is of course a fallacy, because in that little person there has to be a small person who perceives, thinks and makes decisions. And that little person ... It goes on indefinitely, a bit like a Matryoshka doll – a Russian wooden doll that is hollow and contains another, similar doll, that in turn is hollow and that also contains a doll.

The idea of the *homunculus* is also elaborated in the Pixar animated film *Inside Out* (2015), in which the consciousness of the girl Riley is depicted by five figures (five *homunculi*). They are five personified emotions that guide her behavior and experience from an inner control room.

In his book *Thinking Fast and Slow*, Kahneman (2011) describes the two cognitive systems as if they are two distinct characters. He immediately warns the reader that it must be clear that this is a simplification for didactic purposes. In reality, the way our brain works is very complex and cannot simply be reduced to the difference between two discrete minds. To give one example, *system 1* and *system 2* should probably not be considered monolithic systems. In *system 2*, for instance, it is clear that not all processes are conscious and controlled (Evans, 2008). Frankish (2018) notes that explicit thinking in its functioning (*system 2*) should not be completely separated from implicit thinking (*system 1*). Even during explicit thinking, implicit thinking remains present; albeit usually more in the background, although implicit thinking in episodes can still come to the fore during reasoning and thinking.

Also, there are different kinds of *system 1* processes. On the one hand, there are processes that make implicit learning possible: we learn to speak our native language without ever having learned the explicit rules that govern our language, and without the possibility to call to mind the knowledge that we implicitly use (e.g. Reber, 1993). On the other hand, there are processes of *system 1* that have to do with automated behaviour that we have first learned to perform, guided by explicit knowledge, and that we then practised a lot so that after a while its practice does not need our explicit attention or awareness (e.g. leaning to drive a car, to play the piano, to waltz, etc.) (e.g. Klein, 2015).

### Skilled intuition

Although there are some exceptions in the family therapy literature (e.g. Boss, 1987; Keith, 1987), intuition is not a theme that has received a lot of attention. In the broader academic field, intuition is often treated with suspicion. Still, in the wake of the dual process cognitive models, intuition is demystified and resurrected as a theme worthy of scientific attention (Evans, 2010). Kahneman & Klein (2009) for instance studied intuitive expertise produced by *system 1*, and they explain that skilled intuition can be acquired through experience. Such intuition supports the judgments and choices of professional experts in action: they are often unintentionally guided by situational cues that activate a mental model about what to do in that situation. Klein (2003) studied firefighters for instance. Confronted with a crisis situation, rather than considering different possible ways to put out the fire, they immediately – without much reflection – recognize a salient pattern of situational cues and they rapidly respond according to an action script that often proves to be adequate. The more patterns an expert can recognize, and the more extensive his/her repertoire of action scripts is, the more skilled the expert's intuition is. Viewed in this way, intuitive action is the accumulation of learning to recognize patterns and learning to act (Klein, 2003, 2015). There is research evidence that suggests that, at least in some situations, intuitive reasoning may lead to superior decision making (e.g. Dijksterhuis, Bos, Nordgren, & van Baaren, 2006). This refers to situations when a person is confronted with complex, multi-attributed decision problems, like for instance predicting results of soccer matches (e.g. Dijksterhuis, Bos, Nordgren, & van Baaren, 2009). If the person in that situation has a rich history of relevant learning and experience that allows him/her, through implicit processes of pattern recognition, to respond intuitively, such responses seem to be more accurate than responses based on explicit reasoning (Evans, 2008, 2010).

Intuition described as *skilled intuition* (i.e., being sensitive and noticing situational cues, in order to respond adequately to these clues by acting according to specific implicit scripts that one has learned to use automatically) seems to be highly compatible with good family therapy. On the other hand, it must be clear that family therapists should not simply trust their intuition, even though they may be experienced and well-trained: intuition is not very reliable. Therefore, it is best that family therapists use their cognitive *system 1* as a guide to navigate in the session only if it is balanced with the monitoring presence of their cognitive *system 2*. It is optimal if the therapist can flexibly move from intuitive responsivity to explicit reflection and back again. What is needed is that the therapist, attuned to the family's rhythm, can flexibly oscillate between the two systems.

Furthermore, the effect of the therapist's intuitive actions should be evaluated in the light of the feedback of the family members (see chapter 7); their spontaneous feedback in the session, as well as in their feedback after the session obtained by the use of feedback instruments, like the Session Rating Scale (SRS) (Duncan, Miller, Sparks, Claud, Reynolds, Brown, & Johnson, 2003), the Dialogical Feedback Tool (DFT) (Rober, Van Tricht, & Sundet, 2020; Rober & Van Tricht, 2023), or another instrument that systematically invites family members to let the therapist know how they have experienced the session. This is important as research in cognitive psychology showed that skilled intuition can only be learned through repeated experience in environments with reliable feedback (Kahneman & Klein, 2009).

## The dual process of the therapist in action

As we have discussed, dual process theories from the field of cognitive psychology suggest that intuition is the dominant basis for real world decision making and is often effective (Evans, 2010). For a family therapist this means that he/she is supposed to trust his/her intuition in order to responsively attune to the different family members. Intuitive presence with the family members can for instance be considered as a crucial factor in empathic listening, or in what some have called "listening with the heart" (Rober, 2017b). In that sense, the therapist's *fast thinking* can be viewed as a precondition for the development of a sense of interpersonal connection between the therapist and the family members, as well as for the development of a safe intersubjective space in which the family members feel comfortable enough to tell their stories. But being intuitive is also dangerous and can lead the therapist astray if he/she doesn't monitor the effect of his/her intuitive actions on the different family members as well as the effect on the complex therapeutic alliance. Therefore, the therapist has to be a cautious and sensitive self-supervisor, always open to listen to the feedback of the family members and eager to understand such feedback even if it is indirect, ambivalent, or loaded with hesitation.

It could be said that the therapist can be insufficiently responsive in two ways:

- Relying too much on his/her *slow thinking* and not being responsive enough to what happens in the present moment of the session, for instance by remaining an objective observer, by holding on too firmly to one's pre-conceived plans or strategies, by being too faithful to one's model in spite of the feedback of the unique family in the session that they might need something else, and so on. In these examples neither the therapist's intuitive responsiveness or the family's feedback are integrated in the therapist's approach to the family.
- Relying on his/her *fast thinking* in a *reactive* rather than a responsive way (Rober, 2011). Being reactive means that the intuitive actions of the therapist can not be considered as a expression of skilled intuition, but should rather be seen as impulsive reactions aimed at gratifying one's own needs or desires (e.g. one's need to be needed, one's need to feel

useful, etc.) or as the acting out of overwhelming emotions (e.g. fear, impotence, anger, etc.). It may be clear that a therapist who tends to be reactive frequently in sessions might need more training (in order to further develop skilled intuition), or might benefit from some kind of historical/retrospective person of the therapist training or supervision (see chapter 3).

**Towards training and supervision (topics for further reflection)**

If we look at the person of the therapist in family therapy practice using the frame of the cognitive dual process models, this poses the question of *how can this help us to reflect on training and supervision?* This is an important question, but – as this way of looking at family therapy is new – it is probably not yet possible to come up with clear and specific answers. Here I want to give some hints about the directions in which such answers are likely to be found.

Inspired by dual process models, the focus of family therapy training/supervision would be on the flexible integration of *system 1* and *system 2* processes in the session, on the development of the therapist's skilled intuition, and on the promotion of the therapist's self-reflection.

The importance of intuitive reasoning and tacit knowledge is rather underestimated in these times mesmerized by evidence-based medicine (Engel, 2008). There have hardly been any efforts to focus training on what is automatic and implicit in the professional expertise of the therapist. Still, it seems that the therapist's intuitive responsiveness is key to building a good alliance with the family members (Rober, 2017b), and here lies a big challenge for family therapy training: How can we teach our trainees to be spontaneously responsive in the session and trust their intuition? But equally important is the question: How can we teach our trainees to deal with their *system 1* processes in *a responsible way*; by being a cautious and mild self-supervisor, and by using the feedback from the family members and/or a supervisor to do a better job?

As it is, a large part of family therapy training is focused on presenting treatment models (protocols, techniques, etc.) that can help trainees to know *what to do* in family therapy practice. However, as each family is unique and each session is special, we have to teach our trainees also *how to reflect* on what is happening in the here-and-now of each actual session. Therefore, our models should be practiced again and again, in such a way that the therapists' actions become essentially automatic, as they are governed more and more by *system 1*. This will free mental space to, now and then, take a helicopter-view to reflect on what is happening in the session, to notice patterns, to become aware of one's own experiences, and to integrate the implicit and explicit feedback from the family members in ways of approaching the challenges of the session. The therapist needs to reflect on all these things in order to evaluate if the processes in the session are going in the right direction. In that way the therapist's reflecting takes center stage in orienting the therapy process and moving it forward for the benefit of the clients.

## A temporary conclusion

If the therapist at a certain moment in the session notices that he/she didn't succeed in being responsive to the family members, he/she needs to make space for *slow thinking* (reflection). The aim is to correct what was suboptimal in the alliance with the family and to search for responsiveness in a more explicit way, preferably using the explicit feedback of the family members obtained by a feedback instrument. A supervision session can be such a space for reflection in which the therapist's thinking can be enriched by the presence of a good supervisor. However, also during the family session there must be some space for reflection (Flaskas, 2012). Then the therapist is alone and relies on his/her self-supervisory skills. Here we can make the link with the concept of *professional self-doubt* (Nissen-Li et al., 2017): the therapist's self-reflection. Research suggests that *professional self-doubt* is linked with a better therapy-outcome (Wampold, 2017) (see chapter 1). Furthermore, as I will explain in the next chapter, *system 2* can also be linked with the concept of the therapist's inner dialogue (Rober, 2005b).

# 5 The family therapist's inner dialogue

In many ways, inner dialogues are like dreams (Wiley, 2016): everyone has them, but they are vague and unobservable to others, making them difficult to study. In the literature, there is also no consensus on exactly how these inner dialogues should be characterized (Langland-Hassan, 2021). They can only be approached from subjective experiences and introspection. That is why it is good in this chapter to start with a personal story of an event during a family therapy session. The story is about a session with father and Melanie. It illustrates how a therapist talks to himself during a session.

## The story of the session with father and Melanie

We are in the session together: father and his daughter Melanie, 14 years old. It is the first time they come without mother and brother Sam (11 years old). But a lot happened before this session with father and Melanie …

Father had come a long way in recent years, and he had been very down at times in his life. Especially since the birth of the children, things had gone downhill for him. He had become more depressed, and there were more conflicts with his wife because he was very controlling about the way she treated the children. He kept an eye on her, and commented on everything she did. That was very hard for her because he constantly made her feel like she was doing things wrong. He also sometimes left and would come back hours later, but he would not say where he had been.

When he got stuck at work (he is an interior designer and works for a large architectural firm), he was admitted to psychiatry, and it emerged that he had been sexually abused by his mother as a child. He had never talked about it, and he had hidden it away in some deep basement of his mind. However, the birth of the children had rekindled his painful past. He went into individual therapy to try to process his trauma. When that

DOI: 10.4324/9781003458395-9

individual therapy ended, father's therapist referred the family to me for family therapy.

The therapy was difficult at first because father did not trust me. I think he was afraid that I would criticize him and point out the guilt he had towards his family and that he would have to pay in some way for his past mistakes. He was quiet and hesitant. Gradually things got better, especially because of the efforts of mother who was very spontaneous and playful, and thus brought life to the sessions. In the fifth session, father suddenly asked me if he could come alone with his daughter Melanie. His request surprised me, and we discussed the idea together. What would be the benefits of a session with father and Melanie? What would be the risks? It was clear that father wanted to discuss something with Melanie which he found difficult to say when everyone was there. We decided to schedule a one-time father-daughter session, and then continue working with the family.

In that father-daughter session, father said that he regretted the way he had dealt with his daughter Melanie in recent years. He said he had often been short-tempered and easily irritated. He had ignored her as much as possible, because he didn't feel good about being so unloving with her, but he couldn't help it because in that period he had to fight his own demons. "That's why I wanted this session," father said, "to tell her I'm sorry ..."

I had a vaguely uncomfortable feeling and I tried to think about it for a moment. *Irritation*, I realised. It was a vague irritation, I felt, but what was I annoyed about? About father, yes, but isn't it nice that father wants to say sorry to his daughter? *You're ignoring her*, I told father in my inner dialogue. I realized it bothered me that father was addressing me and talking about his daughter, while Melanie sat there and listened. *Why did he tell me he regretted the way he had treated her over the years? He'd better say it directly to her*, I silently contemplated.

Then I addressed father and asked him if he could tell Melanie directly what he had said to me.

"But she heard it, didn't she," he countered.

"Yes, but it means more if you look at her and tell her directly."

I saw that Melanie sat up more. She was getting ready to receive her father's words.

And then it was quiet. I saw him struggling. He didn't look at Melanie and seemed to be absorbed in an inner struggle.

The tension in the session became palpable in my body. I began to doubt. *Did I give him too difficult a task?* I wondered. *No, not too difficult*, I replied to myself, *he will succeed.*

It stayed quiet in the session, but not in my head. *Hang on, Peter, you have to put up with this*, I said to myself. I reminded myself of what I had learned from Minuchin many years ago: *only end the assignment after father has said something and then you have to congratulate him for his courage and his commitment.*

Then father turned in his chair in the direction of Melanie.

*Yes, he will do it,* I exclaimed inwardly.

Father looked at Melanie and said, "I'm sorry, girl. I'm really sorry."

Melanie reached for the tissue papers on the table. Tears ran down her face. She reached for the handkerchiefs, but she couldn't reach them. Father slid the box in her direction. She took a few tissues and dried her tears.

I felt a great relief and relaxation. And my eyes were moist too.

### The inner dialogue

This story illustrates – from the perspective of the therapist – how the therapist, in addition to the conversation with the family members, which is open to everyone, also talks to himself in silence.

We could schematically depict the session with Melanie and her father like this:

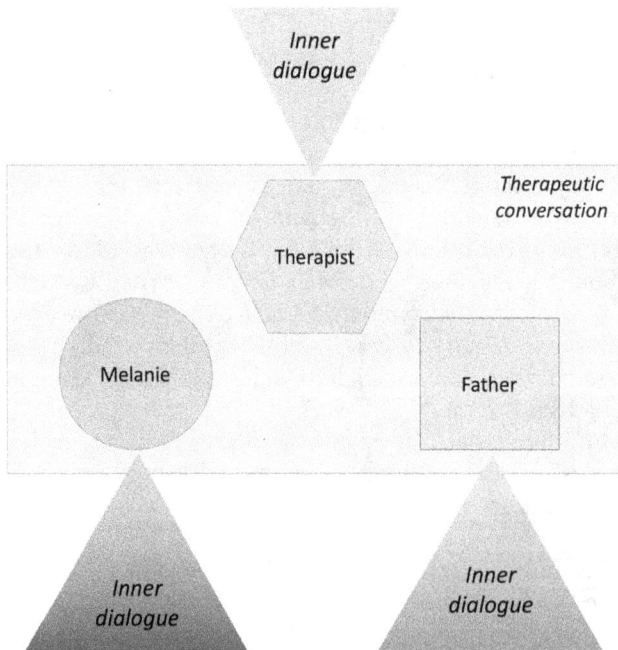

*Figure 5.1* Inner dialogues in the session with Melanie and her father.

It is important to keep in mind that only his/her own inner dialogue is accessible to the therapist. The inner dialogues of the family members are there, but they are by definition inaccessible to the therapist. They are *terra incognita*. Sometimes the therapist, if he/she reads the client's expressions carefully, gets a hint of what is going on in the client's inner dialogue or sometimes the therapist senses things about what might be happening in the client's inner world, but in principle this remains private.

---

**Erving Goffman**

Erving Goffman was a Canadian sociologist (1922–1982) who, among other things, gained fame for his dramaturgical view of the person in everyday life (Goffman, 1959). He states that what a person does in a social context is like a performance for an audience. The person plays a role in which he/she believes himself/herself. This is what Goffman calls *the sincere person*. This is opposed to *the cynical person* who plays a role he/she doesn't really believe in, but that is meant to mislead the public in an attempt to enjoy some benefit to him/her.

For Goffman, the metaphor of theatre is thus very important to analyze the tension between the individual and the social context. We are all actors who play roles in the social arena. There we are on stage doing *impression management*: we show ourselves as we want to be seen and are constantly concerned with the way we are viewed by others. In addition to the stage, there is the *backstage*: that is a space within us in which we keep the things hidden that we do not share with others, or do not *yet* share with them.

---

His/her own inner dialogue is accessible to the therapist. The inner dialogue can even become a very useful tool if the therapist succeeds in engaging the inner self-supervisor as a critical but mild self-supervisor. However, it does take some practice for therapists to become aware of their inner voices. We all have inner dialogues, but we often live as if they don't exist.

### The inner dialogue and the dual process

We can link the inner dialogue to the dual process theories we talked about in the previous chapter. When we just act automatically and intuitively (*system 1*), our inner dialogue does not seem to exist. We blend in with the outside world and play our part. We respond to others: supplement what they say, or oppose their vision and give counterarguments. We encourage others or comfort them or criticize them. We laugh at their jokes; we tell an anecdote, or we offer them something ("Fancy a cup of coffee?"). Our inner dialogue is not central in those moments, because we are primarily concerned with what is happening around us. Our behavior dances along with the people we are in contact with; sometimes we move along, sometimes we go in the opposite direction, but we dance in response to the dance of others.

But there are also times when we stand still, take some mental distance and reflect. Then we withdraw from our interactions with others, as it were, and our attention goes more to our inner world. *System 2* comes to the fore. We are going to explicitly consider things, question them, evaluate them, etc. We think about what we're doing and maybe wonder if we shouldn't do it differently. We set goals and make plans that we divide into steps: first *this*, then *that*, and then *that*. We do these things in our inner dialogue, in which we – like an inner polyphony – talk in different voices with ourselves in silence about how we experience things, what we want to achieve, and how we are going to do it.

---

### The inner dialogue in action

Often, we are not aware of our inner dialogue. But next time you mow the lawn, think about what you are doing inwardly while walking behind the lawnmower. Most likely you are talking to yourself or to inner others. You might talk to one of the kids and explain why you think he/she is exaggerating with their screen time. Or maybe you talk to your mother who died a few years ago and maybe you are telling her about the children growing up. Or maybe you talk to your boss, and inwardly explain to him/her how you would have liked to have decorated your new workspace. You can also hear his/her voice and his/her answer inwardly, to which you respond with counterarguments.

While we are busy doing things, our minds are not empty. No, we have conversations with ourselves, or with imagined others. This is certainly the case with activities that are repetitive and routine, and that we don't have to really focus on (such as mowing the lawn, jogging, driving, etc.). But also, for specific tasks that fully demand our attention (e.g. installing a newly purchased smartphone) we often talk to ourselves. Then our inner dialogue can take the form of self-instructions, warnings, or encouragements.

Therapists talk to themselves, while talking to their clients. You can see that happening in the story of father and Melanie. During the tense silence that arose after I invited father to say directly to Melanie that he is sorry, this is clear: I talk to myself in silence. Let's take a closer look at what I said to myself at that moment. The first voice said *Did I give him too difficult a task?* And then another voice came and said *No, not too difficult*. This second statement is a response to the first statement. This is typical of inner dialogues. One voice evokes the other: sometimes the second voice is a voice of consent but at other times it may disagree with the previous voice. Inner speech is therefore essentially an inner *dialogue*, rather than an inner monologue. Fernyhough (2017) speaks of a *chorus of me*. It is a polyphony: each voice represents a perspective on reality and expresses a view on what is happening or what should be done.

## The self

The *self* is the product of the inner dialogue, with its different voices (Wiley, 2016). It is a *dialogical self* that never finds peace, and is constantly in motion, different voices confirming each other, or correcting and adjusting. One voice evokes the other; as in our example of father and Melanie: the voice that wonders if the task is too difficult evokes a voice to say, *No not too difficult*.

### The inner dialogue in philosophy

According to Socrates – as described in the 4th century BC by Plato (2014) – thinking should be seen as an inner dialogue.

A similar idea can be found in Augustine in the 4th century AD, e.g. in his book *Confessiones*. In it, he shows himself as a forerunner of narrative psychologists when he connects the inner dialogue, his own story, and personal identity (Stock, 2018).

In more recent history, Russian thinkers such as Bakthin, Voloshinov, and Vygotsky have been particularly inspiring for contemporary thinking about inner dialogue.

Bakhtin (1981, 1984, 1986), for example, describes the inner dialogue as if it were a restless pool of different voices: some authoritarian and loud, some soft and peripheral. Some full of emotion, others very firm and rational. Some of the voices represent real existing individuals, but sometimes it's just our own voices, not connected to any real external person, representing our own multiple concerns.

In that way, we're constantly debating with ourselves in silence.

Developmentally, we can say that the inner dialogue, as Lev Vygotsky wrote, arises from external dialogues (which the child witnesses or in which the child is involved). These external dialogues are gradually internalized over a period of months in the first two years of life (Vygotsky, 1962). Just as the child learns to speak the language, so the child also learns to speak to him/herself inwardly. From listening to dialogues of others and participating in dialogues with others, the thinking is kneaded in the form of an inner dialogue.

### Lev Vygotsky

Lev Semyonovich Vygotsky (November 17, 1896–June 11, 1934) was a Russian educational and developmental psychologist.

He is best known for his work on the relationship between language and thought. The prevailing idea at the time was that when the child learns to master language, he/she can express his/her thinking. Language enables the expression of thought, everybody agreed. Vygotsky showed that it is the other way around: the child only really learns to think by developing language.

For Vygotsky, the interaction of the child with his/her social context was central. That may seem obvious, but the well-known Swiss developmental psychologist Jean Piaget (a contemporary of Vygotsky) focused mainly on the development of the child in himself. What Vygotsky saw as a step in internalizing social speech, Piaget called *the private speech* of the child and he saw it as an illustration of the fact that the child did not adapt to the social context in his/her inner communication. He called it *egocentric speech*.

Vygotsky died of tuberculosis in 1934. His work only became known in the Western world in the second half of the 20th century after a few of his books were translated into English: *Thinking and Speech* in 1962 and *Mind in Society* in 1978.

The ideas about the inner dialogue that Vygotsky formulated in the 20s and 30s find a lot of support in more recent psychological research (e.g. Alderson-Day & Fernyhough, 2015).

According to Vygotsky, there is a gradual development of the child from social dialogue to inner dialogue, with the child's *private speech* as an intermediate step. The internalization of speech in the child's development can be represented as follows:

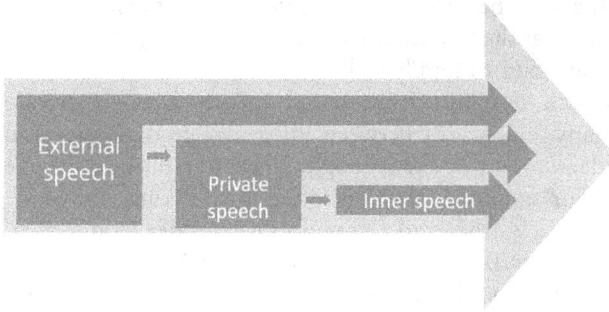

*Figure 5.2* The development of inner speech.

Let's give an example of the child's private speech. According to Vygotsky, private speech develops after the child gets to know the language in the outside world (external speech), so around the age of two to three years. After the child mastered speaking, speaking aloud with himself arises as a possibility for him/her, in addition to speaking with others.

An example:
Thomas sits on the floor and is building a house with blocks. He has already made a high wall and would like to put a few more blocks on top. But the wall is shaky.
"Oops, be careful now," Thomas says to himself.
He takes a block between his thumb and forefinger.
He reaches for the structure with a block but hesitates and withdraws his hand.
"Sit closer," he says.
Thomas moves closer to the structure.
"Be careful, Thomas," he whispers, concentrating.
He slowly brings the block above the wall and gently lowers it.
"Is it going to work?" he whispers.
He places the block on the wall and lets go of it.
"Yes!" he exclaims.
He claps his hands for a moment as if he were applauding for himself.

According to Vygotsky (1962), the most important functions of private speech are self-regulation and problem solving. This is illustrated in the play of Thomas: he speaks aloud to himself in question and answer, as if several children are trying to build a tower together. A child's *private speech* can usually be observed at moments when the child is alone. Sometimes, when others are be present, but not involved in the interaction (e.g. the child is drawing at the kitchen table, while mother is cooking), the child may also talk out loud to him/herself.

Because inner speech develops from social speech through private speech, there are many similarities between inner/private dialogues and social dialogues (Alderson-Day & Fernyhough, 2015; Martínez-Manrique & Vicente, 2015). For example, there is often turn-taking, in which different voices follow each other and respond to each other (confirming, contradicting, nuancing, etc.). We also see this turn-taking in the example of Thomas' private speech while he's building a house with blocks. He asks questions to himself ("Is it going to work?") which he then enthusiastically answers ("Yes!") He even addresses himself by his first name ("Be careful, Thomas").

But inner/private dialogues also differ from social speaking in some areas. For example, inner/private dialogues are condensed and shortened compared to social speech (Fernyhough, 2017). In Thomas' example, we see him saying "Oops, be careful now" instead of "Oops, I have to be careful now." A little later, he says "Sit closer," instead of "I'd better sit closer." These are examples of the condensation of language that can be observed in children who are privately speaking to themselves, but which we also find in inner speech. In the inner dialogue, speaking is more compact, briefer, and faster. Often sentences are reduced to one or a few essential words: the subject of the sentence, and all words related to the subject are omitted. Afterwards, the condensed inner speech can be "unpacked". A statement from the inner speech can be explained in more detail: the person can – with some self-reflection – flawlessly explain what he/she meant by the brief inner comment, and how the statement should be understood in full. Behind the short inner statement, it often turns out that there are much more complex considerations.

### The own language of inner speech

Inner speech differs from social speech: it is shorter, more concise, and faster. But perhaps it is not so different from some forms of social speech. Vygotsky (1962) cites the example of people who are waiting for a bus. The bus is late, and they have been waiting for some time. When they finally see the bus coming in the distance, no one will utter a long sentence like "the bus we have been waiting for for so long is coming". Perhaps it will be more of a condensed statement such as "there it is" or just the naked comment "the bus". After all, the context is clear to everyone and it would be superfluous to make it explicit. Thus, concise speech is not only a characteristic of inner speech, but also has similarities with our informal speech with people we know and trust well, and with whom we share a certain context.

## The functions of the inner dialogue

In the psychological literature on the inner dialogue of the last two decades the inner dialogue is related to many fundamental human processes: language, consciousness, memory, reasoning, and the self (Alderson-Day & Fernyhough, 2015; Langland-Hassan, 2021). Almost all cognitive psychologists who study the inner dialogue seem to agree that thinking is mediated by language, and that the inner dialogue plays a role in these processes. Opinions are divided on exactly what that role is (Langland-Hassan & Vicente, 2018).

Many efforts have been made to map out the functions of the inner dialogue as precisely as possible (Alderson-Day & Fernyhough, 2015; Langland-Hassan, 2021): How does the inner dialogue contribute to the psychological functioning of a person? It is obvious that the inner dialogue is involved in all basic *language functions*: reading, writing, and speaking (Abramson & Goldinger, 1997). Thus, in reading, we will form words inwardly, with rhythm and intonation, even if we do not pronounce the words and we remain silent. Yet inner speech also has an audiological-phonetic quality and is more than pure semantics (meaning). Langland-Hassan (2021) gives the example of sentences with the same meaning, which are "pronounced" differently inwardly in two different languages (e.g. "it is snowing" and "*il neige*"). This is just one illustration, but it shows that inner speech makes a difference in silent reading.

But the inner dialogue, in addition to supporting our reading, also has other, less obvious psychological functions. Overall, research shows that the most important function of the inner dialogue is to support all kinds of complex cognitive processes (Alderson-Day & Fernyhough, 2015; Langland-Hassan, 2021). This concerns important but diverse processes that we can grasp under the general headings of *reflection* (Frankish, 2018) and *self-reflection* (Morin, 2018). This mainly concerns these five functions:

1 *Reflection*: the inner dialogue makes conscious thinking possible (Frankish, 2018). This is an old thought that we already find in Socrates (Plato, 2014), but which is still being elaborated in contemporary psychology. For example, Wiley (2016) puts forward the idea of the dialogical self, to highlight that the dialogue between inner voices is central to our thinking. He emphasizes that this is mainly about practical thinking (*what happens now? What am I going to do? How should I go about this?* Etc.), but that also in abstract or philosophical thinking different inner voices can be in tension with each other.

2 *Self-supervision* or *self-monitoring*: inner dialogue plays an important role in cognitively supporting *executive functions* (planning, monitoring, and inhibiting behavior) (e.g. Frankish, 2018; Morin, 2018). In our inner dialogue we keep an eye on the results of our activities, weigh them against our intentions, and if necessary, we will correct or adjust our behavior.

3 *Developing self-knowledge*: the inner dialogue is a path to self-knowledge in the sense that it helps us become aware of our own thinking (Langland-Hassan, 2021; Frankish, 2018). Morin (2018) states that the inner dialogue is a kind of window on consciousness. The inner dialogue sometimes resembles a continuous voiceover (such as at a sports competition) that comments on what is happening and discusses subjective experiences. Vague thought contents (e.g. experiences, fears, anxiety, etc.) become more clear and aware in the inner dialogue and more sharply delineated so that we can think about them (Bermúdez, 2018). In this way, the inner dialogue contributes to *self-awareness* and being able to think about what is going on in oneself (Morin, 2018). Furthermore, the inner dialogue plays a major role in autobiographical memory. In our inner dialogue, we process our experiences into meaningful memories that together form the story of our lives (Fernyhough, 2017). In this sense, the inner dialogue is very important in the development of our narrative identity and our self-image (Bruner, 2004).

4 *Self-talk*: furthermore, the inner dialogue can also contribute to self-regulation through communication with oneself. For instance, the inner dialogue makes it possible for us to *motivate and encourage* ourselves. This has been studied, for example, in the context of sport[1] in which

---

1 Here – and further in this chapter – we take a brief trip to sports psychology and what is said about the inner dialogue there. It is worth noting that in sports psychology one does not make such a sharp distinction between private speech and inner dialogue (see e.g. Van Raalte et al., 2016, p. 140). Sports psychologists talk about "self-talk" and it doesn't really matter to them whether the athlete talks to him/herself out loud, or in silence. For sports psychologists, the relationship between "self-talk" and the performance of the athlete is much more important than the distinction between private dialogue and inner dialogue (see e.g. Van Raalte et al., 2016, p. 143).

self-empowerment and inner self-encouragement are common, spontaneous, or purposeful (Latinjak, Hatzigeorgiadis, Comoutos, & Hardy,
2019). In addition, especially in more technical disciplines in which fine
motor skills are crucial, self-instruction is also important in sports
practice (Hardy, 2006).

5 *Reflection on selective openness and rehearsal*: not everything that we
silently consider in our inner dialogue we will say out loud. We select
what we say out loud, and how we say it (Frankish, 2018). This happens
automatically when we are interacting with others where we only say
what fits into the flow of the dialogue. However, sometimes we make this
selection very consciously when we explicitly consider whether we are
going to share something with others or not. When we are explicitly
considering what we are going to say, the inner dialogue offers the
opportunity to mentally rehearse what we are going to say (Carruthers,
2018; Frankish, 2018; Alderson-Day & Fernyhough, 2015): we try out
words and phrases in our inner dialogue and we silently hear the voices of
the others who respond to what we said to them internally. This can be
useful, for example, when we are preparing for a job interview or an
exam. This is also very important for the therapist: he/she must constantly
think about what he/she is saying, when he/she says it, and how he/she
says it. Therapists often consider saying something, and then start
rehearsing inwardly, imagining how the client would react. In that
way, therapists choose what they're ultimately going to say and how
they're going to phrase it.

## Reflection on the session with father and Melanie

If we look back at what happened in the session with father and Melanie,
we see that different functions of the inner dialogue come to the fore in the
dialogue. For example, I was supervising myself (function 2) when I
wondered if the assignment was not too difficult for father. There was *self-
talk* (function 4) when I encouraged myself to endure the silence of father's
hesitation and to have trust in father's abilities. The sequence of the
session described begins with the vague uncomfortable feeling. I wondered
inwardly what that vague feeling was exactly and tried to name it.
*Irritation*, I call it in my inner dialogue. This is an example of the 3$^{rd}$
function of the inner dialogue (self-knowledge) and is mainly about
developing self-awareness. After I identified my vague feelings as irritation, there was an inner voice wondering what I was annoyed about. I then
addressed father in my inner dialogue ("*You ignore her*"). I reproached
him for ignoring his daughter by addressing me instead of her, and there
was immediately another inner voice that took on father's defense by
arguing that after all it was nice that he wanted to apologize to his

daughter. I did not express my irritation explicitly (see $5^{th}$ function: reflection on selective openness), but I choose to give father a task and invite him to address Melanie directly. Without making it explicit, I use a therapeutic technique called *enactment* that I learned from Minuchin (Minuchin & Fishman, 1981).

---

**The inner dialogue is not always helpful**

An inner dialogue can be very useful (self-regulation, self-knowledge, etc.) but can also have disadvantages. For example, my inner dialogue can lead me astray if I don't manage to become aware of my real experiences and motives in my inner dialogue (Wilkinson & Fernyhough, 2018). Or worse, sometimes I lie to myself about my experiences, motives, and thoughts. Furthermore, a difference can be made between self-reflection and self-rumination (Morin, 2018). Self-reflection is fueled by a healthy curiosity about oneself and leads to good self-regulation, appropriate self-knowledge, and mild self-evaluation. In self-rumination, self-reflection shoots through into excessive self-focus, panicked doubts, and destructive judgments about oneself.

There is also a lot of research that suggests that the dysfunction of the inner dialogue could lead to auditory hallucinations (Langland-Hassan, 2021). Research shows that with auditory hallucinations (hearing voices), parts of the brain that are responsible for language production are activated, in addition to parts of the brain that are responsible for perception (Allen, Aleman, & McGuire, 2007). The hypothesis is that auditory verbal hallucinations would be the result of the wrong attribution of episodes of inner dialogue: inner voices are assigned to something outside oneself (Wilkinson & Fernyhough, 2018).

---

## Dual process and inner dialogue

The inner dialogue promotes complex cognitive processes of reflection (Frankish, 2018) and self-reflection (Morin, 2018) and in this sense it is not surprising that the inner dialogue appears most explicitly at times when a person functions from Kahneman's cognitive *system 2* (Frankish, 2018): in the explicit consideration of a strategy, for example, in the mental rehearsal of a certain approach to a problem or in the pre-mentalization of a complex movement. Think, for example, of a high jumper who concentrates before the jump and visualizes both the run-up and the jump before he/she starts moving. Frankish (2018) gives the example of a complex calculation task. To perform such a task, I will take pen and paper, and explicitly and intentionally follow a certain procedure in which I divide the complex calculation into several steps of more simple calculations that I can make with my implicit *system 1* (mental arithmetic). In doing so, I will give myself inner clues, question myself, encourage myself, etc. By following the formal procedure step by step explicitly, I can solve the complex calculation task. It is interesting to note that my implicit reflection (e.g. mental arithmetic) is integrated into explicit arithmetic with pen and paper.

---

**Tennis as an inner game**

In 1974, the book *The Inner Game of Tennis* by W. Timothy Gallwey was published, in which the author presents tennis as a double game: there is the game on the court and there is the inner struggle of the tennis player who must overcome uncertainty and nervousness in him/herself. Tennis players perform less well when they take themselves down in their inner dialogue with critical comments and discouraging comments. If, on the other hand, the tennis player tackles his/her insecurity with inner encouragement, it contributes to better athletic performance.

It is also remarkable how Gallwey – who was a tennis coach, not a psychologist – developed his own *cognitive dual process theory-avant-la-lettre* (Gallwey, 1974). He distinguished between *Self 1* which explicitly observes, thinks, and judges on the one hand, and on the other, *Self 2*, which functions automatically and intuitively. It is not difficult to recognize Kahneman's slow system (*system 2*) and fast system (*system 1*) (see previous chapter). Gallwey didn't just recommend the obvious positive self-instruction and encouragement to tennis players, but rather advocated that they let themselves go into the game. Tennis players play best when they give control to the implicit system *Self 2*. While playing tennis, the explicit *Self 1* system must be temporarily sidelined. He refers to D.T. Suzuki's introduction to Herrigel's book *Zen in the Art of Archery* (originally published in German in 1948). In it, Suzuki argues that we come to our greatest achievements without calculation or thought (Herrigel, 1999).

---

The inner dialogue thus comes to full fruition at times when the person functions from Kahneman's cognitive *system 2*. Yet the inner dialogue is also active when intuitive thinking (*system 1*) is at the helm. But then the inner dialogue is less extensive and complex. It is – to use the terms of Vygotsky (1962) – even more condensed, shorter, and faster. In *system 1*, it consists of fragments of associations and impressions, often in the form of short sketchy statements that can be emotionally charged. Drawn-out inner statements and discussions (as with *system 2*) are not in their place in *system 1*, as they might disrupt the automatic and intuitive nature of the action. The quality of a performance in sports, for example, would suffer if one could not let oneself go in the action. The athlete would be distracted by too many inner thoughts.

> For example, the inner dialogue of the high jumper who takes his/her run-up and jumps can consist of very short comments or self-instructions ("faster", "yes, now", etc.), nothing more, because the athlete must be in his/her body, and in the movement.

However, even short inner comments that bubble up naturally during a sports performance can weigh on the athlete's performance, especially if they are discouraging or negative (e.g. "you are so slow again") (Tod, Hardy, & Oliver, 2011). In sports psychology, it is usually argued that the athlete must allow him/herself to let go in his/her movement and in his/her game, unencumbered by any inner comments whatsoever (e.g. Gallwey, 1974). The inner dialogues of a motivational (e.g. "yes, I can do it") or self-instructional (e.g. "keep looking at the ball!") nature should be reserved as much as possible for just *before* the sporting action begins (*system 2*).

## Moments of self-reflection

When a therapist is confronted with a difficulty in the session, or a challenging situation, the therapist will take some time to reflect on what is happening in the session and have an extensive inner dialogue about it – in which *system 2* is in the foreground. In the reflection, the situation is discussed in different voices speaking from different positions, each expressing a certain view. Vague experiences are made clearer, they are labelled and placed in the context. Various options are being considered, often by imagining what would happen if one chose *that* option for action, or *another* (*rehearsing*). In this way, the options are evaluated for their feasibility and effectiveness. In the end, a plan of action is created that seems promising. That plan must then be implemented, but there is often still some hesitation or uncertainty. Then there is a need for encouragement and final advice from inner voices, before one really takes action and surrenders back to the intuitive *system 1*. Yes, it sounds like a team meeting between colleagues, and it looks like it in many ways, but it's a silent dialogue between different inner voices looking for a way to deal with a difficulty.

This is a generic description of how an inner dialogue can proceed in situations where there is enough time that explicit thinking can develop extensively. It is interesting that in such an explicit inner dialogue we work towards implicit thinking: one reflects on the situation and tries to have a plan of action that can be put into practice in small steps that can be taken without thinking. A complex problem is dissected into sub-problems that can be tackled step-by-step through the implicit cognitive system (Frankish, 2018). The therapist must do something with the challenging situation that presented him/her with the dilemma, and at some point, the automatic, responsive system will have to take over again (the explicit polyphony will be pushed back into the background). Once the implicit system is at the steering wheel, the inner dialogue will necessarily be limited to brief encouragements or short comments.

# 6 Emotion regulation of the family therapist

## The Smits family

Following mother's feeling burned out, and with a referral from the general practitioner, the Smits family – mother, Paul, 12 years old, and Frank, 14 years old – decided to go into family therapy.

In the first session, we get to know each other. Mother is a high school teacher. Paul talks about his guitar and about the music class he attends every week. Frank shows me a website on his smartphone about professional cycling, which turns out to be his own website. Mother explains that Frank is a big cycling fan and that he watched cycling races together with his father, mostly on TV, but they had also travelled around Flanders and France to watch some spring classics and the Tour de France live.

"… But now, that will not happen again," says mother.

I ask: "How come?"

Mother explains: "My husband died, about a year and a half ago. He was ill for a few months, then he died. It went pretty fast … Now I have to do it all on my own …"

She gestures with her head in the direction of the children, from which I understand that she is referring to raising the children alone now. I feel pity and also sadness. I think of my wife and see myself standing in tears at her grave. If I lost her, I wouldn't know how to move on with my life.

Mother: "… I miss him so much."

Tears roll slowly down mother's face. I feel the urge to comfort her, and I want to offer her the box of Kleenex. But I immediately ask myself in my inner dialogue: *Do I want to comfort her, or am I looking for a way to try to stabilize my own emotions?*

In discussing this short sequence from my first session with the Smits family, I want to focus on my emotions in the session. I want to focus

DOI: 10.4324/9781003458395-10

especially on what happens to me when mother talks about her husband's death, and how hard it is now to take care of the children alone. At that moment, I felt pity and sadness. On the one hand, I seemed to empathetically connect with mother, but on the other hand I was also catapulted into my own life: an image came to mind of myself standing at the grave of my wife. My attention then jumped back to the session and I felt the urge to comfort the mother by giving her tissues. In my inner dialogue, I wondered what I actually wanted to do: comfort her or balance my own emotions. Maybe I wanted both.

Let's see how the session proceeded ...

Even though I feel the urge to comfort mother, I hold back. *It is not individual therapy here,* I say to myself inwardly, *Mother is not alone.*

I look at the two boys. It strikes me that they sit there motionless and that they do not make any attempt to comfort their mother.

I say: "Paul and Frank, this is a difficult moment. If dad was still around, he could comfort mom when she feels sad. But dad is no longer there. Who is going to comfort mom when she's sad?"

Frank: "Yes, mom often weeps, and then I try to be with her, but I don't know how to comfort her."

While Frank says this, Paul moves his chair closer to his mother, he puts his head on her shoulder and his hand on her arm.

I turn to Frank and I ask: "Sometimes you don't know how to comfort her?"

Frank: "Yes, because sometimes when I try to comfort her, she clings to me and cries even harder."

"Yes, I can imagine that's confusing ..."

I felt the urge to comfort mother, but I did not. On the contrary, I broke free from the emotional identification with mother and turned to the two boys. From my position of emotionally vibrating with the mother, I began to talk with Frank about how he deals with his mother's grief. In this way, Frank managed to talk about his powerlessness, while at the same time, Paul felt the space to exhibit some comforting behavior towards his mother.

The story of the Smits family illustrates the main themes that will be touched upon in this chapter: the emotions of the family therapist in the session, and the way these emotions relate to the complexity of the therapeutic alliance.

### What do we mean by the word "emotion"?

Over the centuries, a lot has been written about emotions, and the connection between body, emotions, and thinking is often questioned.

For example, René Descartes pleaded to separate thinking from the body and emotions: *cogito ergo sum* (I think therefore I am). In the wake of Descartes' ideas, rationality, untainted by emotions, was seen in Western thought as the highest good. At the end of his life (in 1649), Descartes finally decided to write a book on emotions, *Les Passions de l'Âme*. In it he stated that emotions are related to physical reactions (e.g. changes in blood circulation), that the soul suffers the influence of the body. In order to protect the independence of our thinking we have to learn about our passions and find ways to control them.

The mind-body relationship is also central in William James' ideas about emotions in classic *The Principles of Psychology* (1890). According to James, emotions are connected with autonomous bodily reactions. Our body reacts *before* we sense our emotions: when we encounter a bear in the forest, our body reacts (heart rate increases, we sweat, etc.) and we flee before we realize that we are afraid.

In 1994, Antonio Damasio's book *Descartes' Error* was published. He explained the *somatic-marker* hypothesis: there are somatic signals that are connected to emotions, that guide behavior and choices. According to Damasio, Descartes made the mistake of detaching thinking from emotions.

In a lot of traditional research on emotions, it was assumed that the emotions have evolutionary origins, and that each existing emotion has contributed to our species' survival in its own way. It was assumed that emotions are biologically anchored, genetically determined, and therefore universal. More and more, however, it is clear that emotions are also socially and culturally determined. For example, Gergen (2009) talks about emotional scenarios: an emotion doesn't only refer to an experience, but it can also be seen as a *performance* according to social rules. Emotions are things we do with others. Mesquita (2022) builds on that idea of emotional scenarios, arguing that emotions are largely culturally determined. Not only the way we express them, or how we deal with them, but also the emotions themselves are permeated by culture. Depending on the culture in which we grow up and live, we experience different emotions. This challenges the traditional view that emotions are *inside us* and closely connected with our bodies – in our heart, in our belly, in our brain. According to

Mesquita, emotions happen *between us*, in our relationships, families, communities, cultures. It's something we *do*, together with others: "like partners in a dance, your emotions and those of others complement and steer each other to form the interaction" (Mesquita, 2022, p.164).

In line with the work of scholars such as Gergen and Mesquita, I will have a broad view of emotions in this book: they are relational and culturally situated. Emotions are about what a person experiences in relations with others (feelings, moods, stress, etc.) and how a person deals with it together with others. Emotions are systemic and dialogical (Bertrando & Gilli, 2015): they emerge out of our relationships and are enacted together with others.

## Emotions

When considering emotions in psychology, scholars often refer to general models of emotions. For instance, there is Magda Arnold's model in which she focuses the *appraisal* of the situation as a crucial factor in the emergence of emotions: for example, in a situation that I evaluate as threatening, I will feel fear. For this reason, Arnold's model is called the *appraisal theory of emotion* (Arnold, 1960). Another theory is the *two-factor theory* of Schachter and Singer in which not only the evaluation of the situation (factor 1), but also the physical arousal (factor 2) is said to contribute psychologically to the experience of an emotion (Schachter & Singer, 1962). In the present chapter, we will work with the model of Mikulincer and Shaver (2016), which further elaborates on the two-factor model of Schachter and Singer.

Mikulincer and Shaver's model states that emotions proceed in four steps:

1 The person perceives a change in his/her internal or external world. This can be a positive change (e.g. a success) or a negative one (e.g. a threat).
2 Automatically, that change is evaluated and generally appreciated as positive and desirable, or as negative and undesirable. This process is called *appraisal* and it results in a specific emotion, depending on the context, expectations, goals, etc.
3 Automatically, a physiological response is triggered, as well as a tendency to action.
4 This then leads to the experience of the emotion and to the expression of the emotion in behavior, thoughts, facial expression, etc.

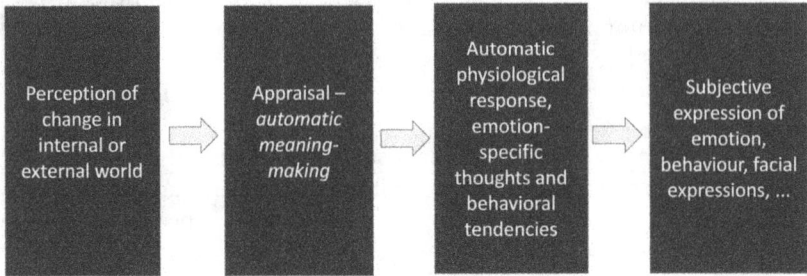

*Figure 6.1* The emotion model of Mikulincer & Shaver (2016).

So, the subjective experience of the emotions only emerges in the fourth step of the model. In the three first steps there are changes that the person undergoes of which he/she is not aware. In the best case scenario, they can be reflected on retrospectively.

### Emotion regulation

In principle, there is a tendency to go through these four steps when a meaningful change takes place in an individual's situation (especially when it is unexpected or unannounced). However, it could be that the emotion or its expression is undesirable because of social norms (e.g. at a funeral certain emotions are not appropriate), for the sake of self-protection (e.g. I do not show my vulnerable emotions if I think others would make fun of me), or for other contextual reasons. Emotion regulation is the process we use to influence what we feel, when we feel it, how we feel it, and how we express it (McRae & Gross, 2020; Gross & Barrett, 2011).

Overall, emotion regulation can be said to intervene in any of the four steps of the emotion process (McRae & Gross, 2020; Gross & Barrett, 2011):

1 We try to avoid threatening situations, or if we do end up in such a situation, we try to leave that situation as soon as possible or try to change the situation. Furthermore, we prefer situations that are not threatening and that evoke positive feelings.

2 *(Cognitive) reappraisal*: we try to look at the situation we are in differently in order to exert some influence on our emotional response, or we focus our attention on something else in our situation than that which evokes our uncomfortable emotions.

3 We try to influence our physiological responses (e.g. by doing relaxation exercises).

4 We can suppress the expression of the emotion (e.g. we can be anxious but pretend not to be), or only partially express the emotion (e.g. only

show a sad facial expression, but when asked why we are sad, deny that we are). We can also feign an emotion (e.g. feign joy when we are actually disappointed).

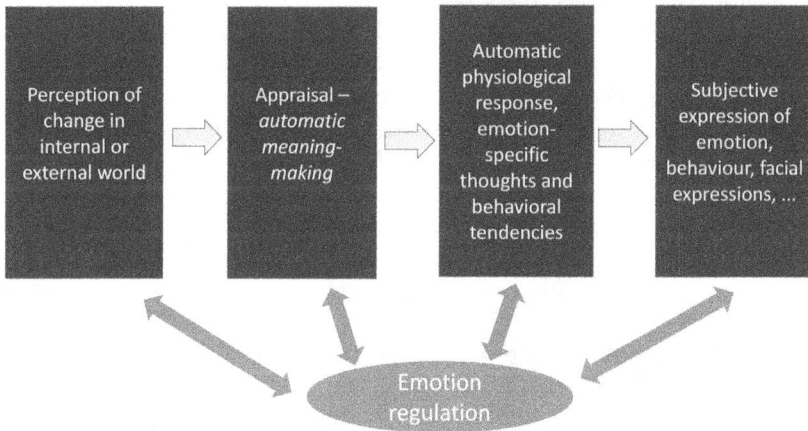

*Figure 6.2* Emotion regulation model.

## Emotion regulation and attachment

Emotion regulation from a developmental psychological perspective begins immediately after birth. When a baby feels threatened (pain, hunger, strong noise, etc.) he/she displays attachment behavior (for example, he/she starts to cry), and a responsive parent is thereby mobilized to remove or reduce the threat. The first emotion regulation we learn is therefore of a social nature: as a baby, we cannot yet regulate our own emotions, but our emotions are regulated with the help of sensitive and responsive parents (or other care figures). "(T)he attachment system is, in itself, an emotion regulation device" (Mikulincer & Shaver, 2016, p. 188). Such emotion regulation can be called *co-regulation*.

Besides co-regulation, there is also *self-regulation*, which is a form of regulation learned gradually by the child. An important step is the evocation of mental representations of care figures, also called *object constancy* (Mahler, Pine, & Bergman, 1975), or *object permanence* (Piaget & Inhelder, 1966). Other major steps in the child's development (learning to walk, learning to talk, etc.) also contribute to the child's ability to regulate his/her own emotions. In adults, self-regulation sometimes happens implicitly and automatically, but it can also occur more explicitly through the inner dialogue (self-talk for instance, in which someone encourages him/herself to overcome nervousness or fear).

An example: a mother says that she received a phone call from the school director who reported that her son Floris (11 years old) was not yet in the classroom that morning, and it was already 10 am.

"Is Floris sick?" asked the school director.

He wasn't sick. He had left home that morning with his bike as he does every morning. After she put down the phone, mother was overcome by anxiety. She tried to calm down by breathing deeply (she had learned that in yoga class), so that she could think clearly (*self-regulation*). Then she decided to call her husband. He remained calm and listened to her.

He suggested: "Let's wait and see, and if Floris hasn't shown up at 11am, I'll come home, and we'll figure it out together."

The conversation with her husband had brought her some peace because she felt that she was not alone (*co-regulation*). When she put the phone down, the ring tone immediately sounded again. It was the school director who called to reassure her: Floris had arrived. He had witnessed a traffic accident on the way to school and had been questioned by the police. As a result, he had only arrived at the school at a quarter past ten. He had a note from the police that confirmed his story.

### Emotion regulation in psychotherapy

Emotion regulation is important in psychotherapy. It is one of the therapist's tasks to help the clients regulate their emotions (Soma et al., 2020). After all, clients often struggle with emotions; sometimes because the emotions overwhelm them (e.g. a client is having an anxiety attack), and sometimes because they control their emotions in a cramped or rigid way (e.g. avoiding emotions by rationalizing, or by avoiding situations that may trigger difficult emotions).

At times when a client experiences emotions in the session, the therapist will work with those emotions in the here-and-now of the session. If necessary, he/she takes on a kind of homeostatic role: when an emotion rises too high in the client, the therapist will try to help bring the emotional tension down again to a level that is comfortable and livable. The therapist can use various specific techniques for this (e.g. breathing exercises), but usually the therapist will also invite the client to talk about his/her experience. The intention is that dwelling on emotions, labeling emotions and connecting those emotions with experiences and events from the client's life, help him/her to get a better grip on his/her emotions and to regulate them. This usually works, provided that the therapist listens empathetically and provided that he/she can authentically convey that the experience of the client is understandable, given what the client has experienced.

Specifically in family therapy, there is the additional fact that family members share emotions not only with the therapist, but also with each other. What the son says about his emotions is heard by mother and father, and it will evoke something in them. The daughter's tears do not leave the other family members cold. Mother's anger affects everyone. And so on. This makes family sessions so difficult, as the family members are – compared to individual sessions – more reluctant to show emotions because of the presence of the other family members. But it also makes family sessions very powerful, because emotions expressed in the here-and-now will trigger something in everyone. When in a family session an emotion needs to be regulated, it is best that the therapist holds back and looks at how the other family members react. While in an individual session a therapist may immediately choose to take up the homeostatic role, in a family session there needs to first be a moment of watchful waiting in which the therapist leaves room for the family's own homeostatic processes. After such moments in which the therapist can observe the family's emotion regulation, it is interesting for the therapist to reflect with the family about what just happened, and to make the family's emotion regulation a topic in the session.

There is another specific possibility a family session offers, in comparison to an individual session. The family therapist can invite a family member to address someone directly when they experience something in the session: "Can you explain to your son how you feel?" "Can you tell your father what you are going through?" "Can you address your mother and tell her what you're experiencing right now?" and so on. This can lead to very intense moments in the session. Just think back to the story of father and Melanie (chapter 5) in which father was invited to address his daughter to say *sorry* to her directly. Such moments are exciting for the family members, but also for the therapist who must bear the tension that is aroused by the *enactment*. Such moments of direct sharing of unspoken experiences are also very therapeutic in the sense that they often lead to a deeper emotional connection between the family members.

The emotion regulation in psychotherapy is not limited to the client's emotions. The emotions of the therapist are also touched in the session and must be regulated. This may be surprising to some, because often one expects the therapist to be an objective professional who is not touched by what happens in the session. That image is wrong. After all, it is important that the therapist is present in the session with the family. The therapist should not strive to be objective and unaffected but should really participate as a subject in the dialogue with the client. He/she must *be* a therapist, with an emphasis on the word "be". In the psychotherapy literature one speaks of *presence* (Hayes & Vinca, 2017): the therapist is fully present as a human being; involved in what happens in the session and what happens does not leave him/her cold. If the therapist is really with the client, then it is inevitable that he/she is emotionally touched, and that is crucial. After all, being emotionally touched is the basis of the therapist's empathy and in that sense, it contributes to the result of therapy (see chapter 1).

It is true that the emotions of the therapist also entail risks and may counteract the effect of therapy. Such risks have to do with the strength of the emotions as well as the nature of the emotions. If the therapist's emotions are too strong (e.g. very strong sympathy with a client's grief) this can hinder the therapeutic process. Furthermore, certain emotions (e.g. irritation) are more difficult than other emotions (e.g. pity). After all, some emotions are in tension with the therapeutic aspirations of empathetic listening, authenticity, and hopefulness (Muran & Eubanks, 2020). The risk of openly expressing some emotions (anger, for example) is that they could lead to a break in the alliance, or make it difficult to build a good therapeutic relationship and create insecurity (e.g. cooperation becomes more difficult, distrust in the relationship, etc.).

---

### The emotions of the therapist and the hesitations in the family

In individual therapy, dealing with the so-called *resistance* of the client (as family therapists we prefer to call it *hesitations*; see Rober, 2017b) is very important (Muran & Eubanks, 2020). Research shows that therapist are often not aware of the resistance of their clients (Hara et al., 2015). It also appears that the emotional reactions of the therapist to the resistance of clients makes a difference in the effectiveness of the therapy (Westra et al., 2012): dealing positively and understandingly with resistance leads to the best result. If the therapist reacts negatively (e.g. defensive, irritable, anxious, etc.) this may strengthen the resistance (Westra et al., 2012).

In family therapy work with adolescents, for example, the hesitation (especially in the beginning of therapy) often lies with the adolescent (Escudero & Friedlander, 2017). The adolescent then says things like "I don't have a problem" or "there's nothing wrong with me". The tendency might occur to the family therapist to draw the adolescent's attention to the things that are not going smoothly in his/her life, and that there are always things to work on. The therapist could also try to motivate the adolescent by pointing out the opportunities that family therapy offers for a happier coexistence in the family. It is unlikely that such intervention will convince the adolescent to engage during the session.

Clinical experience has taught us that these types of interventions do not work and on the contrary often lead to more negative interactions with the adolescent (distrust, reluctance, etc.) in which the family therapist then threatens to get caught up. A *split alliance* may be developing in this way. In such situations, feelings of irritation and powerlessness often arise in the therapist.

It is better to approach the adolescent's hesitation differently. The family therapist must find a way to deal with the adolescent's hesitation empathetically and acceptingly. For example, the therapist may choose to make room for the adolescent's stories about his/her good reasons to hesitate (Rober, 2017b). Often hesitations in the session are connected with disappointing experiences concerning past attempts to cope with the difficulties (e.g. conversations with professional helpers, discussion in the family at home, etc.): "we talked to the family doctor about this but he blamed me", or "we tried to discuss this at home but my mother started to hyper-ventilate", etc.

By dealing with hesitations in the right way, the family therapist can avoid being involved in an escalating emotional spiral with the hesitant family member and from sinking into negative emotions (powerlessness, irritation, fear, etc.) himself/herself.

## What about the therapist's emotions in the session?

The general rule is: the therapist should fully experience the emotions evoked in the session, and at the same time he/she should try to ensure that the alliance with the family members is not compromised by his/her emotions. Sometimes the therapist can even do more than just protect the alliance. For example, it could be that the therapist can use his/her emotions to better understand the family members, or to strengthen the alliance and promote safety in the session. I will explain this in more detail below.

The starting point of dealing with the therapist's emotions in the session revolves around these 2 basic ideas:

1 *Emotions have an important function in the development of the therapeutic relationship.* For example, part of the communication of the family members takes place through the experience of the therapist. If the therapist wants to listen carefully to the client's story, he/she must not only listen with their *ears* but also with their *eyes* and *heart* (Rober, 2017b). What the therapist experiences during the session may also tell

a part of the story of the family members. He/she must carry and bear his/her experience, instead of internalizing (avoiding, pushing away, suppressing, etc.) or externalizing the experience (acting out, reacting, etc.).

2 *The regulation of the therapist's emotions in the session is important* for several reasons:

1 So that the emotions do not take the therapist out of his/her therapeutic role (empathy, acceptance, etc.), and so that the development of a safe therapeutic relationship is not compromised.
2 So that they can be used to better understand family dynamics (this is *listening with the heart*; see Rober, 2017b).
3 So that they can be used in the development of therapeutic interventions that are better tailored to the family members and where they are in their processes by considering the therapist's own experiences in the session.

As mentioned earlier, many authors in the field of emotion regulation distinguish between self-regulation and co-regulation (Mikulincer & Shaver, 2016). This distinction has been beneficial, but when we focus on the emotion regulation of the therapist in the family session, self-regulation and co-regulation prove difficult to distinguish. In a family session, processes of co-regulation of emotions are continuous and complex. Because of the way family members interact with each other and with the therapist in the session, they are constantly implicitly (and sometimes also explicitly) regulating each other's emotions.

### The story of Carina and her family

It is the first session with the family of Carina (16 years old) who was raped a few months ago when she returned home after school on her bike. She had not taken the shortest route, but had instead taken a longer way back home in the hope of meeting a boy she was in love with. However, she encountered a man who pulled her off her bike and raped her.

In the session Carina says:

"Ah, it was ultimately my own fault. I had no business in that neighborhood. I should have gone straight home after school."

I feel inner protest. I want to contradict her and assure her that rape is never the victim's fault.

But before I can say anything, mother intervenes: "It's not your fault, baby. You couldn't help it."

My experience changes instantly. A sense of relief is washing over me, and I no longer feel the need to intervene and tell Carina that she is not to blame.

I feel open to listening to Carina's story as she addresses her mother: "That's true, mom, I couldn't do anything about it. But I've learned my lesson. I will stay away from that neighborhood. It is never going to happen to me again."

The example of the session with Carina and her family illustrates an implicit process of co-regulation in a family session. Carina's statement that it was her own fault that she was raped evoked strong emotions in me. The emotions were resolved when the mother in response emphasized to her daughter that it was not her fault (it is worth noting that the mother said exactly what I wanted to say). This situation exemplifies the general statement: *people in dialogue continually regulate each other's emotions.* While such emotion regulation is real, it is not an intentional process. It is rather something that is experienced by the participants (family members and therapist) over the course of the session, and it usually remains unnoticed (although sometimes therapists do notice it in retrospect, for instance when they watch the video of the session).

### The self-regulation of the therapist

In addition to the co-regulation experienced by the therapist in the session, a family therapist can also try to regulate his/her emotions him/herself. This can be done in several ways, and we can, inspired by McRae & Gross (2020), specifically distinguish five self-regulatory strategies a family therapist can use:

1 *Avoid situations in which the emotions could be evoked.* An example: a therapist has sexual problems in his personal relationship with his partner and he feels very insecure. In the therapeutic sessions, even though he mainly does couple therapy, he avoids the theme of sexuality. He never takes the initiative to discuss sex with his clients.
2 *Fleeing the situation in which the emotions are evoked.* For example: a therapist feels that the family session is moving towards a theme that is potentially very conflictual in the family, and that scares her. She has always been conflict-avoiding, and she now also steers the conversation away from the conflict by giving a psycho-educational explanation about solving problems in families.
3 *The therapist does not allow himself/herself to acknowledge the troubling emotion because he/she is focused on something else in the*

*situation.* For example: though the therapist did not feel it during the session, when watching the video recording of the session afterwards, he recognizes the powerlessness that he had not allowed himself to feel in the session.

4 *Self-supervision* and *self-talk*. For example: the tension in the session rises and an argument threatens to erupt between a father and his 18-year-old son. The therapist feels his own anxiety creeping up on him and tells himself: *stay calm now, relax now.*

5 *Reappraisal* (also called *cognitive restructuring* or *reframing*). For example: a therapist has learned to reframe tense family situations as a challenge, rather than as a threat. This helps her to remain present as a therapist in threatening situations.

We can now take a closer look at these five strategies.

It is usually inappropriate for family therapists to avoid certain themes because of their own discomfort (strategy 1). Fleeing from a situation is usually also not recommended (strategy 2). Furthermore, it is advisable for the therapist to pay attention to the issues that are important for the family, notwithstanding his/her own discomfort (strategy 3). Yet every family therapist sometimes falls back on these kinds of unproductive strategies to regulate his/her emotions in the session. Although this is not best practice, therapists are still human and these kinds of mistakes happen from time to time.

Self-supervision (strategy 4) has many functions, and emotion regulation is one of them. A therapist who feels discouraged can encourage him/herself. A therapist who feels threatened by concerns from his/her own personal life can remind him/herself to focus on the session. A therapist who is in danger of drowning in the despair that prevails in a family might advise him/herself to instead look for signs of hope. And so on. Self-supervision always presupposes a kind of self-observation: the therapist observes him/herself (*what do I do?*); listens to him/herself (*how do my words sound?*); and is aware of his/her experiences in the session (*what do I feel?*). Such self-observation can then, for instance, lead to *self-talk* (e.g. encouragement) or *self-instruction* (e.g. reminding him/herself to be empathetic towards each family member).

The most researched self-regulation strategy is *reappraisal* (strategy 5) (McRae & Gross, 2020), which is usually referred to as *reframing* in family therapy (Newsome, Mitchell, & Awosan, 2018). Although it is a technique of self-regulation, it can also be applied in the session to help the family members view their situation from a different angle. This technique is initiated by the therapist, who must first reassess the situation, attaching a more positive or hopeful perspective. Only if the therapist can reframe the situation for him/herself can he/she try to convey the reframing authentically and credibly to the family members. Reframing works best if the therapist can concisely present to the family members a new and surprising perspective on what they are going through – one that is more hopeful, or that better validates the commitment of the family members. If a reframing is successful, it often leads to a feeling of relief and relaxation, initially in the therapist, and then also in the family members. This is illustrated below in the case of Amy and her mother.

### Amy and her mother

It is the first session with a single mother and her daughter Amy (15 years old). Mother says that she is raising her daughter alone because her husband (Amy's father) died 10 years ago.

"Died?" I ask.

"He committed suicide," mother says.

A little later in the session, mother tells me that Amy told her last week, on Boxing Day, that she has been cutting herself. Amy had told her mother: "I started cutting myself in the summer. Especially on my legs. I cut until it bleeds and then I stop."

As I listen to mother's words, it evokes sadness in me.

Amy is silent while her mother talks, and I have the impression that she is ashamed.

Mother is in tears and says: "Apparently Amy's been cutting herself for months, and I hadn't noticed. Am I a bad mother?"

I feel mother's despair. *How terrible it must be for a mother for this to happen without her noticing.*

"I don't want to be a bad mother," mother continues, "and I haven't had a good example myself. My mother was never home. Always at work."

I remind myself that it's always difficult to try to be a better parent than your own parents have been. It's easier when you have had a good example that can inspire you as a parent than when you have had a bad example that you desperately want to avoid replicating.

"I want the best for my child. I don't want her to hurt herself," mother says. "I'm besides myself. What should I do?"

She begins to cry.

Amy sits in silence. I don't see that shame anymore that I thought I saw a few moments ago. She looks like a sphinx, who is emotionally unaffected by what is said in the session. I, on the other hand, feel that mother's hopelessness is closing in on me. She had just asked *What should I do?* and I realize that I don't have an answer to her question. I feel powerless. In my inner dialogue, I try to encourage myself: *stay calm. Don't be intoxicated by mother's despair. And try to keep listening to what is being said.*

I focus on the conversation, and mother tells me that she is especially angry with herself because in recent months she had tried to be more present for Amy. She had noticed that her daughter was struggling with something: Amy had had a big conflict with her best friend over the summer because they were both in love with the same boy. Mother was also alarmed because Amy was retreating to her room more than she used to. She watched one Netflix series after another, and she did not say much when they were together (e.g. at dinner). Fortunately, Amy continued to do well in school, which reassured mother a bit. Still, mother sometimes wondered if Amy might be depressed, as her father had been for years before he committed suicide. That is mother's biggest fear: that also Amy would commit suicide. As a response to that anxiety, mother had been trying to make more time for Amy in recent months. She had started working fewer hours and tried to do more things with Amy.

"But Amy wasn't very excited about my attempts to connect," mother says in the session.

And then Amy protests: "But I went to the movies with you in November and we hiked in the woods together on Christmas Day."

Amy's input gives me hope. Not necessarily the content of what she says, but mainly *that* she says something. And then suddenly, I realize that I had to look at Amy's conversation with her mother on Boxing Day differently. Yes, Amy had delivered a painful message ("I cut myself until it bleeds"), but more importantly, for the first time in months, she had confided in her mother about something she had been hiding until then. Mother's attempts to make contact with her daughter after the summer had apparently made room for something new. I feel my despair melt away completely as I realize that I can authentically complement mother on her efforts the past few months.

I say, "Perhaps because you were more present with Amy, she found the courage to share with you that she was cutting herself. That is an important step forward!"

In this case, I was first swept up in mother's despair, and mainly use self-talk as a self-regulatory strategy ("*stay calm*"). Then, sparked by Amy breaking her silence, I came to the realization that there is another possible interpretation of the conversation on Boxing Day in which Amy talked about her self-injury for the first time. Amy (finally) talking to her mother about it is a sign that trust is growing between them and that she is confiding in her mother more. By looking at the conversation between mother and Amy differently, I was able to regulate my own feeling of despair, which in turn made a difference for mother, who felt relief after hearing the therapist's reframing.

The story of Amy and her mother can be seen as an example of the emotion regulation of the therapist by *reappraisal*. But it is also an example of the complex relationship between self-regulation and co-regulation. The helplessness that descended upon me in the session was regulated by Amy's unexpected contribution. This contribution sparked hope in me, providing a fertile ground for nurturing my later self-regulating *reappraisal*.

## Intentional co-regulation

In some circumstances, the family therapist can also actively choose to involve others in the regulation of his/her emotions. This is an important approach because the regulation of the therapist's emotions can also be beneficial to the family members (for example, by helping the family members to regulate their own emotions) and additionally contributes to the development of a safe and effective therapeutic relationship.

This process of intentional co-regulation consists mainly of inviting the family members to talk about certain experiences that the therapist selects, based on his/her own emotions in the session (Byng-Hall, 1995). This has to do with the vibrating of the therapist's sensitive string (see chapter 3). The unspoken question driving the therapist is: *what about the family has made my sensitive string vibrate?* The point is that the therapist needs to find a way to talk about this emotion without putting him/herself and his/her own experiences center stage in the session. The therapist uses his/her emotions in the session, but the main idea is to use them to make space for the emotion of the family members and for the sharing of their experiences. In his/her inner dialogue the therapist can explore how his/her experiences in the session might fit into the family's dynamics. This technique can be called *emotion reflection*. It is illustrated in the next case.

### The case of Tina and her parents

In a family session, Tina (a 16-year-old) says that she contacts boys and men via Tinder. She then sometimes meets them somewhere at a café. When I hear this, I feel anxiety bubbling up in myself. Tina then talks about an experience with a man who suggested that she go home with him. She had flirtatiously said "no" to that proposition, and the man had not insisted.

I feel uneasy, and in my inner dialogue I say: *I'm worried. This kind of situation could easily go wrong.* I think about it for a moment and realize that my anxiety, if it continued to grow, could threaten my therapist role. Indeed, my anxiety could become so great that there would be no room for anything else. For example, the anxiety might infect me to only see Tina as a girl who does dangerous things. and in that way my interest in Tina as a person might be suppressed. I decide to try to do something with my emotions.

I ask Tina, "I feel worried about what you're saying about Tinder and those guys and stuff. Can you tell me something that can reassure me?"

Tina laughs and says: "You're like my parents."

In my inner dialogue I tell myself: *Tina is giving me the feedback that I listen to her from the position of her parents.* I have to free myself from that position to be able to have a broader perspective on Tina. I don't really have to think about it, and I immediately know what to do.

I turn to the parents and ask: "Does Tina have a point there? Are you worried about her?"

The parents nod and talk about their anxiety and how they are trying to help Tina be more careful and take some precautions.

I feel my anxiety subside immediately, and I feel that I can listen more openly again. I can now speak to Tina and her parents about their life together from a better position: free from the anxiety that narrowed my view, and open to whatever else is there in the family.

In this short example of the session with Tina and her parents, we see how I take the initiative to do something with my experience in the session in such a way that my worries become regulated through the family members. In this way I can listen more openly and work with the family from an optimal position. This case also illustrates how the emotions evoked in the therapist are often a reflection of emotions that are present somewhere in the family, but that have not yet been expressed in the session. This is also illustrated by the following case.

### The case of Lucas, Eva, and their parents

Lucas (six years old) is a very anxious boy who also has sleeping problems. Lucas comes together with his sister Eva (ten years old) and their parents for a first family session. At the beginning of the session, it becomes clear that the parents are on the verge of divorce (father has been living apart for two months), and that they are now – because of their concerns about Lucas – together in one room for the first time in a few weeks. From the beginning of the session, there are enormous tensions between the parents, and I feel that it is not impossible that an open conflict could arise in the session.

Despite the tensions, I try to get to know them, and this part of the session goes all right. But then we talk about the worries they have about Lucas' fears and then they start to blame each other for Lucas' difficulties.

Father says in a soft tone:

"Yes, growing up is not easy and every child sometimes struggles with nightmares of course, but if you are treated as an infant and smothered in kindness, you do not learn to deal with fears."

Mother replies:

"Well, and when a child sees his father having outbursts of anger, that doesn't help either."

In this way they send each other reproaches and I feel that this threatens to lead to open conflict. I try to mediate a bit more by rephrasing the words of one in ways that hopefully are more acceptable to the other, but I feel it doesn't work. I feel powerless. I notice that I am also afraid of the conflict. In my imagination, these people can go very far in their hostile behavior, and I want to avoid that here in the session, especially in front of the children.

I look at the children for a moment, and I notice that Eva has moved her chair closer to Lucas' chair. She also has put her arm around his shoulder. Hey, I hadn't noticed that a moment ago. That must have happened when I tried to manage the conflict between the parents.

I ask the parents to be quiet and listen for a while, " ... because I would like to talk to the children."

The parents sigh, but they say it is ok.

I address the children: "Lucas and Eva, I see that you are sitting closer together now than at the beginning of the session. That's beautiful, and I wonder, Lucas, did you move your chair in Eva's direction or did you, Eva, move your chair in his direction?"

Eva replies: "I saw that Lucas was getting scared. And then I moved my chair closer to him. And then I comforted him."

"Nice," I say. "And is that what you do at home when there are conflicts between mom and dad?"

"Yes," Eva replies. "That's usually in the evening when we're already in bed. And then I crawl into bed with him."

*So the parents try to save up their conflicts until the children are in bed*, I say to myself in my inner dialogue. *Good idea, but the children are not fooled and know full well what is going on between you.*

"Mmm, so then you crawl into bed with Lucas," I say warmly. "It's hard for kids when their parents can't get along anymore. It scares them, and perhaps also it makes them powerless."

I mentioned being afraid because I knew from the registration form that Lucas was struggling with fears, and I mentioned powerlessness because I had felt that myself earlier in the session when my attempts to mediate proved futile.

"Yes," says Eva, "I often feel powerless and sad, because I haven't been able to make sure my parents are happy together."

"In what ways have you tried to help them?" I ask.

I talked to the children for another 20 minutes, while the parents listened. The tension between them was gone. They were worried about the children, and they asked to come the next session without the children, to talk about the impending divorce. I turned to Lucas and Eva and asked what they would think if their parents came without them.

"We think that's a good idea," Eva said.

"They like the idea," I said to the parents, "nice, and yes, me too, I think it might be a good idea."

We made an appointment for the next session.

In this case, my emotions were like a reflection of what the children felt: fear, insecurity, powerlessness. Because I addressed the children out of an awareness of my own experiences, there was empathy for Lucas' fears and recognition for Eva's efforts. It is often beneficial for the family therapist who is burdened by certain emotions in the session to ask him/herself the question: *how would these emotions that I now feel so strongly fit into the family dynamic?* If the therapist succeeds in discussing similar emotions to those he/she experiences with the family members in the session, things that were previously left unsaid can become part of the dialogue. In addition, the therapist will be relieved to find that he/she is free from his/ her emotional burden.

### Utilizing one's own experiences in the session

If the therapist wants to deal responsibly with his/her own experiences during the session, it is advisable to follow these 3 steps:

*Step 1.* Awareness by focusing:

In step 1, the central question the therapist asks him/herself is: *What do I feel? What am I experiencing?*

I must focus on my experience and try to get a clear picture of exactly what I feel.

---

**What exactly do I feel?**

Sometimes I immediately grasp what it is exactly that I experience. But most of the time it's not that easy because what I feel is differentiated and complex. Then there is exploration in my inner dialogue about what I experience exactly. Typically, different voices mention different things that are in play. Each of these voices highlights a part of my experience, but there is no voice that fully grasps it. It is important that I consider the complexity of that inner discussion and accept that my feelings are differentiated and cannot be captured with one label.

Often I do not manage to focus satisfactorily on my experience during the session – there is often little time to think in the session. Then I must think about it further after the session. It can help if I can talk to someone about my experience: a colleague or a supervisor. Talking about what you went through can clarify what it meant to you.

What sometimes helps me to get a clear picture of what exactly I am experiencing is to ask myself what my feeling would make me do if it took complete control of my behavior. When I think about that question, I am usually confronted with grotesque fantasies of things that I would never really do, but that magnify my feelings so much that it sometimes makes clearer what exactly is at play.

It is also important to consider that I may be experiencing secondary emotions (Greenberg, 2010). These are emotions that are a reaction to other emotions. For example, it could be that I feel irritation, but that this irritation is actually a reaction to the powerlessness that is evoked in my work with the family. We call this powerlessness *a primary emotion*. The irritation then is a reaction to the powerlessness, and it is called *a secondary emotion*. Secondary emotions are often easier to bear than primary emotions. They usually put the pressure outside of ourselves and are less threatening to us. For example, it may be less difficult for me to be irritated with a family member than to feel that I am not making any difference and that all my efforts to help the family are in vain.

*Step 2: Reflection on the possible link with the family's dynamics:*

Here is the central question for the therapist: *What can I learn about the family from what I experience in the session?*

The starting point is the idea that what I experience as a therapist during the session has to do with a sensitive string in me that is vibrating (see chapter 3). The string is in some way connected to my personal history, but the fact that it has started to vibrate in my contact with *this family* can provide important information about the family. That is why it makes sense to dwell on questions such as: *How do my emotions fit into the dynamics of the family?* Even if I have just had an inner discussion about my experience during the session, I can reflect on the question: *In what way do my different inner voices reflect differences between family members?* I ask myself these questions, and I hope that in my inner dialogue there will crystallize something that will help me to understand the family better. I usually can't find complete clarity in my inner dialogue, but I often find enough clarity to take the next step: thinking about promoting dialogue with the family.

### Step 3: Reflection on promoting dialogue with the family:

Here is the central question: *How can I use my experience to advance the therapeutic process?*

As a therapist, I want to make room for experiences of family members that have not yet been put into words in the session in order to advance the therapeutic alliance. The exploration of the place of the therapist's own experience in the context of the family session can take the form of a *co-reflection* with the family: this is a process of metacommunication in which the therapist enters a dialogue with the family about the course of the session (Muran & Eubanks, 2020), and thereby also tries to give his/her own experience a place. Rather than offering a therapeutic interpretation or an explanation to the family, it is an invitation to the family to explore together what is actually happening in the session. The therapist can say something like "Let's stop for a moment, and think about what is happening here now … what is it like for each of you to be here in this conversation now?" Then usually a hesitant process begins in fits and starts. Everyone must switch from *being in* the process to a kind of meta-position from which they *reflect on* the process and on their own experiences. Everyone is searching for words that can express what they are experiencing. It is crucial that the therapist participates in such a metacommunication conversation from a position of authentic *not-knowing* (Anderson & Goolishian, 1992). He/she has to be open to answers that are new and surprising to him/her. On the part of the therapist, it should certainly not be a quest for reassurance or for confirmation of one's own vision.

The therapist is focused on guiding the search process with the family for the meanings that play in the session, but at the same time he/she is feeling how his/her experience fits into the image about the dynamics that gradually emerges in the conversation. This is often an exercise in *multidirectional partiality* (Boszormenyi-Nagy & Sparks, 1973), in the sense that the therapist listens empathetically to everyone's story without losing sight of his/her own experience. The different experiences of the different family members are all pieces of a jigsaw puzzle, and they sketch a whole together, but the experience of the therapist is also a piece of the puzzle that has to fit in one way or another. Sometimes out of this process with the family an image emerges that seems to be right for everyone. Sometimes that doesn't work, and important questions remain unanswered. These questions are then considered further in the process. Perhaps there will be clarity later. What such a co-reflection does in any case is to regulate the emotions of each of the family members: everyone reflects on their own experiences and looks for ways to talk about those experiences. Everyone is listened to by the others, and – if everything goes well – empathetic responses are shared.

### Hannes and his family

Hannes is an 18-year-old boy who comes to family therapy with his family. He has been depressed for a while and has had a short admission to youth psychiatry. Now he is back home but the psychiatrist advised them to go to family therapy after discharge.

In addition to Hannes, the family also consists of Charlotte (21 years old), father, and mother.

It's the first session. During the first minutes I get to know the different family members a little bit: father is a jazz musician who plays in a band, but mainly teaches in Brussels' music academy. Mother has a luxury clothing store. Hannes is in the last year of high school and studies mathematics and sciences. Charlotte is in the third year of the bachelor's program dance at the Antwerp School of Arts. Music, dance, and visual arts are important for all family members, except Hannes. He is only interested in Instagram and Netflix.

After getting to know the different family members, I ask who is most worried in the family. All family members look at mother. Mother notices this and says that she mainly wants peace in the house, and that she hopes that family therapy can help in some way.

Father replies that he does not know whether family therapy is useful for them.

"Is it always good to talk about things?" he asks rhetorically. "I don't know. What you don't talk about doesn't exist."

Charlotte then says: "In our family, we never say *'let's talk about it'*. Things are hanging up in the air."

Father goes on to say: "Yes, and Hannes doesn't want to talk with us and that weighs on the family. He shuts himself off completely and does not accept any help from us. He doesn't see that we might be able to give him good advice. In the end, we have more life experience and wisdom, don't we?"

Hannes is quiet and he radiates that he does not intend to say much in this session.

I'm trying anyway: "What could this family therapy mean for you, Hannes?" and as I hear myself asking this question, I already feel that it will lead nowhere.

Hannes doesn't look at me when he says: "I wouldn't know."

Mother says: "It's hard to get through to Hannes. I don't know if I understand him. I don't know if anyone understands him." Mother sighs.

I feel a lot of tension. *A minefield*, I think to myself. *A minefield in which the words can explode at any moment, and in which it may be safer not to speak.*

I let the silence weigh for a moment and then decide to try a co-reflection.

I say: "This conversation has been going on for 25 minutes now, but what is actually happening here? What's going on? What's it like for you to be in this conversation?"

It's quiet for a moment.

I say: "Yes, let's be quiet for a moment to feel what we feel, and clarify what we're thinking."

I leave a silence.

Then I ask: "Who wants to start by saying something about what's happening here?"

Charlotte says: "For me as a sister, it's hard to see that Hannes is unhappy. He doesn't say it, but he radiates it. I'm afraid he doesn't have anyone to talk to, and I sympathize with him."

Father picks up on it: "I find it worrying that Hannes doesn't talk."

I answer: "But you asked yourself a few minutes ago if it always makes sense to talk about things?"

When I hear myself say this, I become aware that there is a pinch of irritation in the way I say this. I hope father didn't hear it. I realize that I have to be careful that I connect with him sufficiently. *Listen to him*, I say to myself in my inner dialogue, *try to understand him.*

And while I give myself this advice in silence, father answers my question: "Yes, I do wonder if speaking is always useful, but Hannes exaggerates. As a father, surely you're allowed to expect a little respect from your own son?"

I reply: "Yes, indeed, respect is important in a family."

I try to connect with father with these words and I notice from the short nod with his head that he feels heard.

Mother says: "I would like to have more contact in the family, without conflict or tension. It seems that we just can't do that."

I try to summarize it a bit and say: "So, in essence, what happens here in the session is what also happens at home. There are many things that are not said. These things are not said out of fear that there will be conflict? Do you think I understand what's going on?"

Everyone nods in agreement. Hannes makes a cautious head movement, I notice. For the first time, I also have eye contact with him for a fraction of a second. For the first time I have the feeling that Hannes allows me to be present as a therapist. It encourages me to move on.

"So speaking is dangerous in your family? It's a minefield?" I try.

I consciously use the metaphor of the minefield, which earlier bubbled up naturally in my inner dialogue.

Again, consent.

I continue: " ... and it seems to me that that is especially difficult for you, Hannes. That is why it may be good that you keep silent in this session. Don't step on a mine ... I hope you have someone to talk to ... someone you can talk to safely, without having to be afraid of explosions and conflict ... "

I continue to talk quietly, looking at Hannes, but without expecting an answer from him. I now speak out of my attunement with him, and I pay attention to subtle bodily signals that guide me in my talking.

" ... Maybe you have a good friend who listens to you. Or an uncle or an aunt ... "

Then Hannes breaks the silence: "I have my therapist ... I can talk to her. I don't need them." He makes a head movement towards his mother and father.

"Oh," father says indignantly. "I find that a frighteningly worrying statement now. We are the parents, but we don't know that therapist and we are not allowed to contact her ... "

I intervene: "Here it happens again. You, Hannes, take the risk to speak and that leads to conflict because you, dad, feel disrespected as a father. You want Hannes to accept your help, because you can see that he is struggling, but he rejects your help. He wants to stand on his own two feet. And you, Charlotte, are a little bit on the margin of it all, but you are very involved, and you empathize with everyone. You understand your parents, but you also understand Hannes. You are pretty much the home therapist of your family. "

I say this last sentence jokingly and it works.

There is a bit of chuckling and there is some relaxation in the session.

The session continued for a while. I mainly tried to understand the different positions of the family members as well as possible. Furthermore, I was focused on making everyone feel that I understood them.

In the next session, this process continued, often laboriously, until something unexpected happened. I didn't see it coming, but Charlotte suddenly said there was something important they hadn't talked about yet.

It became quiet in the session, and I felt the tension rise.

Charlotte continued, "Yes, we don't normally talk about it, like it didn't happen, but it did happen."

Silence.

Then Charlotte said: "We actually have an older brother, James. Four years older than me. But he committed suicide a few years ago."

I was completely surprised. They hadn't said anything about it in the first session, but I remembered again the words of father who said that it is not always necessary to talk about everything. Now it turned out that they had kept their son's suicide quiet all the time.

I gently asked: "May I ask you to tell me a little more about James and his suicide?"

"Well, we suspect it was suicide," mother said. "He overdosed on drugs."

Mother then told the story of James, who always had a hard time growing up. Things didn't go well at school. He didn't follow the rules and had bad friends. He was involved in thefts. At the age of 14 he started experimenting with drugs. First it was weed. He later became addicted to heroin. Mother had made many attempts to talk to him – "James was mommy's darling," Hannes added – but James went his own way and got lost in life, until it proved fatal to him. Mother's story also revealed that father had not been worried about James during that period. "It'll be fine," he had appeased when his wife wanted to talk with him about James. After James' suicide, father had started to reproach himself a lot, and he has felt deeply guilty. When the difficulties with Hannes later arose, he certainly did not want to make the same mistake and tried to be there for Hannes. It was baffling to him that Hannes did not accept his help.

The therapy with Hannes' family is a long story (which fortunately ends well in the end), but I wanted to tell it here to illustrate how co-reflection with the family, based on the therapist's own experience, can work. It is crucial that the therapist focuses well on his/her own experience, and then invites the family to do the same. In addition, the therapist must attune well with each of the family members, even though their stories may be very different and sometimes they may even contradict each other.

## The discomfort of the therapist as a compass

A family therapist can use his/her discomfort during the session as a compass, including his/her dissatisfaction, his/her concern, his/her fear, his/her shame, etc. Whatever he/she may feel during the session, the family therapist needs to reflect on what he/she experiences. While it is his/her personal discomfort, it is being evoked at present during the session with this family. Carefully considering his/her discomfort can therefore point the family therapist towards themes that are important to discuss with the family.

To use his/her emotions as effectively as possible in his/her therapeutic actions, it is helpful for the therapist to feel an appropriate level of comfort in the session. If the therapist feels *too comfortable*, he/she is not touched by what is said in the session. If the therapist feels *too uncomfortable*, he/she mainly experiences stress, which can cause the therapist to focus on self-preservation and self-protection. It is optimal if the therapist feels *appropriately* or *slightly uncomfortable* in the session.

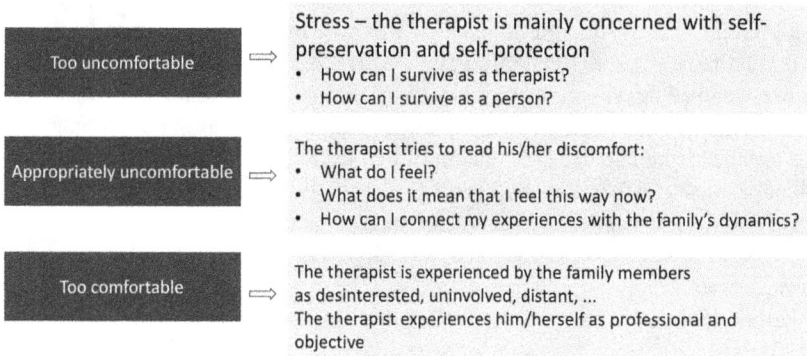

| Too uncomfortable | ⇒ | Stress – the therapist is mainly concerned with self-preservation and self-protection<br>• How can I survive as a therapist?<br>• How can I survive as a person? |
|---|---|---|
| Appropriately uncomfortable | ⇒ | The therapist tries to read his/her discomfort:<br>• What do I feel?<br>• What does it mean that I feel this way now?<br>• How can I connect my experiences with the family's dynamics? |
| Too comfortable | ⇒ | The therapist is experienced by the family members as desinterested, uninvolved, distant, ...<br>The therapist experiences him/herself as professional and objective |

*Figure 6.3* Emotions and the therapist's comfort.

Feeling *appropriately uncomfortable* means that the therapist senses as a person (more than as a professional) that something is not right for him/her, and he/she is not completely at ease. If that is the case, then his/her experience can be optimally used in the service of the therapeutic process. The therapist can dwell on his/her discomfort and try to understand it. Through focusing on the discomfort and trying to verbalize it, the therapist can reflect on ways his/her discomfort can be useful for the therapeutic process. In this chapter, I provided several examples of a therapist who used his discomfort therapeutically. This happened, for example, in the session with Tina, that 16-year-old Tinder user, in which the therapist used his anxiety as a theme of the questions he asked the girl and her parents. It also happened in the session with Hannes' family, where the therapist discussed his experience that the session might be a minefield with the family. And it also happened in the session with Frank and Paul with which I started this chapter: the therapist used his own experience as a stepping stone to talk with them about comforting their mother.

# *Stairway to heaven*: Jason Sonck and his family (part 2)

The therapy with Jason and his parents was two months in progress.

It was halfway through the fifth session. Jason hadn't said anything yet, his silence weighed heavily on the session, like dark menacing clouds. It seemed as if the raging storm could erupt at any moment. I understood Jason's silent anger. It was unfair that he had to be the victim of that terrible accident. His life had been full of promise and then it was all gone. Suddenly. Without cause, without guilt. A stupid accident, it happened in a few seconds.

I looked at mother. She seemed sad. She was about to cry. I sensed her powerlessness.

Father looked at me and said, "I don't know if you understand how it feels … "

He didn't finish his sentence.

I thought I understood. I am a father myself and my son is also a guitarist. I could sympathize with father. Maybe I understood him too well. By thinking about it for a moment, I realized that – like father – I too actually wanted to keep Jason alive. I also realized that that might be a problem. I wondered: *How can I be a good family therapist for this family if my feelings are with the parents, rather than with the son?* I also realized that in the past few sessions I had tried to compensate for this imbalance as much as possible, by generously empathizing with Jason's suffering. I let him talk about what happened to him, how unfair it was that he lost everything that was dear to him. I listened intensely and I hoped he had felt heard. Later this would prove to be a vain hope.

Father explained that there had been a lot of conflict in the last week. The reason was that Jason had gone to talk to grandma, father's mother. Jason had gone to explain to the old woman that he wanted to die. He hoped she would understand him. Grandma was happy at first that she could be there for Jason, until she understood that he had come to her because he thought that her life with all those old age ailments was also meaningless and that she would be better off dead.

DOI: 10.4324/9781003458395-11

Grandmother was completely upset and called dad: "Do you think I should be dead?"

Father immediately drove up to her to calm her down.

When he returned home later, he sought out Jason.

A big argument ensued and then a days-long menacing silence in the family that extended into the session.

"I don't know if you understand how it feels ... " father said.

"I don't know if I understand either," I said, "but tell me how it feels to you ... "

Father talked about his concern for his mother who had a very difficult time seeing meaning in life after her husband's death. One time he went to visit her after work, and when he rang the doorbell, no one opened the door. He thought that was strange and he was worried. He let himself in with the key, and he found her in bed.

At first, he thought she was sick.

She just didn't feel like getting up. "Why should I?" she had said.

"That touched me deeply ... " father said, " ... and then Jason does something like that ... "

Silence.

"I understand that you're angry," I said, "and I understand from you, Jason, that you were looking for someone who understands your sense that life has lost meaning."

Jason remained silent, but in the way he looked at me I thought I saw a flicker of recognition. Maybe I had found some connection with Jason after all.

However, I couldn't think about it because father went on:

"Yes, I understand Jason feels alone," dad said, "I understand." Then he turned to Jason and said, "But what I what I can not understand is that you want to be dead. Your mom and I gave birth to you. We've always loved you. We took care of you, changed your diapers, fed you with the bottle, we guided you through your first steps and we were so proud when you said your first words."

Father turned to me: "If you love your child, if you watch your child grow up, if you're proud of your child because he's wise and talented ... Then it is not conceivable that he would be dead. You just don't want to think about that."

I listened and I couldn't help but think of my own child. My son. How he grew up; with good days, and bad days, but mostly with good days. I remembered a dramatic moment when we were very worried that he would have an incurable illness. There were worrying symptoms and we saw that the doctor was also worried. She suggested additional examinations. Only after a few months and several intensive medical examinations did it become clear that there was nothing to worry about. I saw it before my eyes again, but now I had to be with this family; with Jason who wanted to die and with his father who wanted him to live.

I said: "I think I understand that as a father, you want the best for your son. From the beginning when he was a newborn, and even now – even though he has had this terrible accident and may have to bear the consequences all his life."

I uttered those words, but in my words also echoed my emotions and the old grief associated with my own son and those tense weeks when we were terrified.

I saw that my words brought peace to father.

He was silent and relaxed.

But Jason, he suddenly stood up – jerky and laborious, but without hesitation.

"I'm o-o-o-off," he said, and he stepped toward the door.

"Jason?" I said, surprised.

"There's no point in this f-f-f-f-fucking therapy," he said, and he walked to the door.

He took the door handle in his hand and turned around, "For me, the therapy is f-f-f-f-f-finished," he said. And then he addressed me, and he said without stuttering, "And you, you're the worst therapist in the world."

He opened the door, stepped out into the hallway, and slammed the door behind him with a dry smack.

# Part III

# Becoming more effective as a family therapist

# 7 Feedback orientation of the family therapist

As I mentioned in chapter 1, based on years of psychotherapy research with *randomized controlled trials* (RCTs), we can conclude that psychotherapy works (Barkham & Lambert, 2021) and that the quality of the therapeutic relationship is the most robust predictor of therapeutic change (Norcross & Lambert, 2018). The most important advice for practicing therapists seems to be: connect empathically with the client, be flexible, and avoid *one-size-fits-all* therapies. The therapist must be willing to be open to the client's feedback and to tailor the therapeutic relationship to the needs and preferences of the specific client (Norcross & Wampold, 2019).

In the past decade, there has been a movement in the psychotherapy field towards integrating client feedback in psychotherapeutic practice (Lambert, 2010; Lambert & Shimokawa, 2011). Several authors have recommended that practitioners invite patients to give feedback on their experiences in the session (Lambert, Whipple, & Kleinstäuber, 2019) using simple and short questionnaires to collect the feedback at the end of each session. Scientific evidence has shown that the use of client feedback can increase the effectiveness of psychotherapy (Lambert, Whipple, & Kleinstäuber, 2019). For example, it leads to a reduction in the breakdown of therapy and to a better dose/effect ratio (e.g. Shimokawa, Lambert, & Smart, 2010). If the therapeutic relationship is difficult, the therapist can use the client's feedback to gain deeper insight into what is causing the difficulty and thus take steps to adjust the therapy and restore the relationship (Norcross & Wampold, 2019). Furthermore, research suggests that incorporating client feedback increases their motivation and empowerment (de Jong, et al., 2014).

---

**More realistic expectations**

At first, feedback-oriented work seemed like the holy grail of psycho-therapy. The first studies suggested that therapy would be much more effective (Anker, Duncan, & Sparks, 2009; Lambert & Shimokawa,

---

DOI: 10.4324/9781003458395-13

2011). These high expectations have been reduced to more realistic proportions by later studies (Lambert, Whipple, & Kleinstäuber, 2019).

Feedback-oriented working does not always lead to an improvement in effectiveness. A study in a psychiatric emergency department in the Netherlands found no effect of feedback-oriented work on the effectiveness of treatment (van Oenen et al., 2016). In a study in Norway, they did find an effect, but that effect was much smaller than the effect that one would expect from the first studies (Amble, et al., 2015).

Nevertheless, overall, research continues to find a positive effect of feedback-oriented work on the effectiveness of therapy (Lambert, Whipple, & Kleinstäuber, 2019; Barkham et al., 2023), and based on that research, the systematic use of client feedback by therapists is recommended.

Feedback-oriented work is not only useful because the effectiveness of the therapy is promoted by optimizing the therapeutic relationship, but, perhaps even more importantly, it also ensures that the therapist learns and improves (Wampold & Owens, 2021). By working in a feedback-oriented way, the therapist is invited to reflect on him/herself, which has been indicated in previous research to help the therapist gradually become more effective (Miller et al., 2020; Blow et al., 2023). Rousmaniere (2017) considers a feedback-oriented approach to be an important part of what he calls *the path to expertise.*

It is important to mention that the effect of a feedback-oriented approach is achieved not through the feedback instrument itself, but through its user (Prescott, Maeschalck, & Miller, 2017). As Chow (2017) succinctly phrases it: "it is the user of the tool, not the tool itself, that influences client outcome" (p.327). For example, some therapists benefit more from client feedback than others: therapists who are more open to the client's feedback make better use of it (de Jong et al., 2014). Such openness has to do with a focus on what surprises in the feedback and what can be learned from it. Effective therapists are not looking for a reassuring confirmation of what they already thought or of what they hoped to achieve in the feedback of clients. Rather, they are looking for what they did not expect or where their good intentions did not lead to the desired result. With this information, they try to do something constructive (Chow, 2017). This also implies that a feedback-oriented approach is primarily effective when the therapist is *receptive*, i.e. open, and curious about what the client wants to share. Furthermore, the therapist cannot learn anything from feedback that is positive but general (e.g. "it was a good session"). Especially critical and detailed positive feedback are useful. The client's feedback should make the therapist reflect, leading to what some have called *professional self-doubt*, which refers to the reflective questioning of the therapist's own actions (Heinonen & Nissen-Lie, 2020). Such reflection on oneself as a therapist seems to be correlated with good outcomes, at least if it is self-critical but also mild: *love yourself as a person, doubt yourself as a therapist* (Nissen-Lie et al., 2017).

And then it is up to the therapist to be responsive: to do something constructive with the clients' feedback. A first step should be to talk with the client about the surprising feedback: being curious and inviting the client to explain his/her perspective in more detail. Here too, the therapist must be strong enough in his/her shoes so that he/she does not feel the need to justify him/herself or to explain what his/her good intentions were. The therapist should therefore not react defensively, but rather he/she should be grateful that the client takes the risk of giving honest feedback. In that way, feedback-oriented work can contribute to a good exchange between the therapist and the clients, and to the client feeling that he/she is really listened to. This is very important: the strength of feedback-oriented work does not lay in taking questionnaires or in measuring effectiveness, but rather in the proper use of the client's feedback to optimize the therapeutic relationship.

Considering the feedback from the family members does not in any way mean that the client is in control and directs the therapy. No, the therapist remains at the helm of therapy. It does mean that the therapist is curious and listens to the perspective of the different family members, and that he/she talks to the family members about their own – and hopefully surprising and possibly critical – perspectives. In addition, it is often the case that the different family members each put their own accents in their feedback, and it is even more rule than exception that they contradict each other. Then it is important that the therapist enters into a conversation with the family to try to clarify the different positions of the family members. Through such a discussion the therapist will better understand the experiences of the different family members, but the family members will also begin to understand each other better. The intention is also to reflect together with the family about the way in which the therapy best proceeds. In doing so, the therapist shows that he/she considers the perspectives of the different family members in the choice of direction, pace, themes, etc. for the next sessions. In this way, feedback-oriented work contributes to building trust in the relationship and so the different family members also receive recognition: they feel heard, notice that the therapist is really interested in them, and experience that the therapist bears them in mind. They also experience how the therapist deals with the differences between the family members that surface through feedback-oriented work: the therapist acknowledges everyone's perspective and looks for a way to move forward together that takes into consideration as much as possible the different perspectives that are present in the family.

## Being feedback oriented as a family therapist

Considering the complexity of the therapeutic relationship in family therapy, the feedback orientation of the therapist is likely to be a crucial factor in working with families (Lappan, Shamoon, & Blow, 2018; Karam & Blow, 2023). However, working in a feedback-oriented way as a family therapist is challenging for several reasons. One reason is that many of the traditional feedback tools that have good empirical support in terms of reliability and validity were actually not developed with the complexity of the therapeutic alliance in family therapy in mind (e.g. the OQ45, the ORS). Rather, they are tools that have been developed for use in individual therapy. While it is possible to use these instruments in family therapy, the family therapist usually encounters the limitations of those instruments rather quickly. This is why we (Karine Van Tricht and myself) have developed our own instruments, with the conjoint setting of a family therapy session in mind (Rober, 2017b; Rober, Van Tricht, & Sundet, 2021; Rober & Van Tricht, 2023).[1]

---

### Our feedback tools

In our work with families, we have experimented a lot to develop our instruments. We started in 2011 using existing questionnaires (OQ 45, CBCL, ORS, SRS, etc.). We soon learned that the proper use of feedback tools presupposes that you create a feedback culture with the clients (see Rober, 2017b): a context in which clients feel safe enough to also give critical feedback. Furthermore, in that period we also asked our clients what it was like for them to work with these instruments. From that survey it emerged that our clients found it useful but according to them many of the instruments we used were too extensive and too cumbersome to fill in after each session. It also bothered them that the questionnaires often asked for things that were not related to the concerns that had brought them to therapy. For example, lists of complaint or symptoms (e.g. CBCL) are sometimes used as feedback tools. Such lists consist of dozens of items that must be scored after each session. *That is very cumbersome,* our clients told us. This made us understand that a feedback tool should be brief. We set the limit at max. five questions. *It also must be relevant,* our clients told us, *we don't want to have to score session after session items that we know*

---

1 Our various questionnaires can be downloaded for free via the website: www.intherapytogether.com.

*from the beginning are not relevant to us.* Based on that feedback from our clients, we then developed feedback tools that we thought would be useful in the therapeutic work with families. We started using these instruments, and we refined them over the years until we came up with instruments that we came out with in 2014.

## The Dialogical Feedback Questionnaire (DFQ)

The Dialogical Feedback Questionnaire[2] (DFQ) (see Attachment 2) is mainly developed for use in therapies with families with children (six years old or older), adolescents, young adults, and adults (Rober, 2017b). It is a simple tool that assumes that the family members who fill it in are sufficiently comfortable with reading and writing.

The questionnaire is completed by each family member at the end of the session and inquires how the family members experienced the session. This is done through five specific questions:

1  Did you tell us what you wanted to say in the session?
2  Have you felt understood by the therapist?
3  Have you felt understood by your partner/other family members?
4  What surprised you during the session?
5  What touched you during the session?

These are open questions and then for some questions the family members are asked to give a score on a scale of 1 to 10.

I refer to my previous book (Rober, 2017b) for a more detailed discussion of the DFQ. Here I want to illustrate the use of the DFQ in family therapy using a case, specifically the case of Alex and his parents.

In my description of this case, I have focused on some meaningful sequences of interactions between the family members and the therapist to illustrate that it is interesting to systematically make room for the feedback from the different family members and that the DFQ can be a useful tool for this. While it may not be possible to be completely a-theoretic, an instrument like the DFQ can be used across family therapy models because it focuses on common therapy factors (especially the therapeutic alliance).

---

2  We used to speak of the Dialogical Feedback Scale (DFS), but because it is actually not a quantitative tool, we now see that it is better to call it a *questionnaire* instead of a *scale*.

*Alex and his parents*

Alex is 19 and an only child. He attempted suicide a few weeks ago, and then was hospitalized in a general hospital to recover from his wounds. There he was visited by a psychiatrist who spoke with him and with his parents. The psychiatrist referred them for family therapy.

*First session*

"Life is a story that ends badly. In the end, the hero dies."

He said it with some hesitation, but without a trace of irony. I couldn't help but think of Albert Camus, and I thought it was charmingly worded for a 19-year-old.

His father probably thought otherwise. He sighed deeply and turned his eyes away. He seemed annoyed.

"Yes, that's how life is ... in the end there is death," I said, and I hoped that with those words I could connect with the son, without irritating father too much.

"We love you, Alex. We don't want to lose you," mother said.

She had tears in her eyes.

Alex shrugged.

*Don't his mother's tears touch him?* I wondered.

"It will happen someday," he said quietly, "but first I want to finish my book."

"Finish your book?" I asked.

"Yes, I've been working on a novel for a while."

I heard father sigh, but I pretended not to hear it and continued talking to Alex.

"Tell us a bit more about your book."

Alex hesitated, but then moved on.

"It's almost done. Well, actually, it's done. But every time I reread it, I start to tinker with it again."

"Is it because you are not easily satisfied? Or ... "

"Yes, I set my bar high."

"What do you mean? Where is your bar?"

Another hesitation on Alex's part before he continued.

"Actually, if I'm honest, I want it to be an international bestseller. That's the goal. So my book must be very good ... "

I didn't taste an ounce of irony in Alex's words.

I looked at father. The irritation was visible on his face.

And with mother I mainly saw sadness: tears and a handkerchief with which she tried to stop the tears.

The session was coming to an end, and I suggested to the family members to fill out a feedback questionnaire. I gave each a blank copy of the Dialogical Feedback Questionnaire (DFQ).

While the family members were filling out the questionnaires, I tried to summarize the session in my inner dialogue. Alex had been struggling with life for several years, in ups and downs. He had moments when he was very optimistic and full of confidence. Then he had big plans and he wanted to push boundaries. But maybe it was those big plans that got him into trouble. He would be disappointed, and then he would become depressed and feel deeply insecure. Yes, the referring psychiatrist suspected bipolar disorder, and from what I had seen in the session, I understood that she was thinking of that diagnosis. The parents tried to help Alex as much as possible, but it seemed as if mother had given up. She seemed to be pulled down deep in her sorrow. Father, on the other hand, seemed mainly irritated and angry. I felt a vague tendency to want to protect Alex from the anger of father. I should probably not do that. This was the question I asked myself: *How can I make room for father's anger, and still make sure Alex isn't destroyed by father's fury?* I noticed how I used big and fierce words in my inner dialogue, while I hardly knew these people yet. *Slow down, Peter*, I said to myself. *Wait for the feedback questionnaires.*

After the session I took a look at the questionnaires.

Here's how Alex filled out the DFQ:

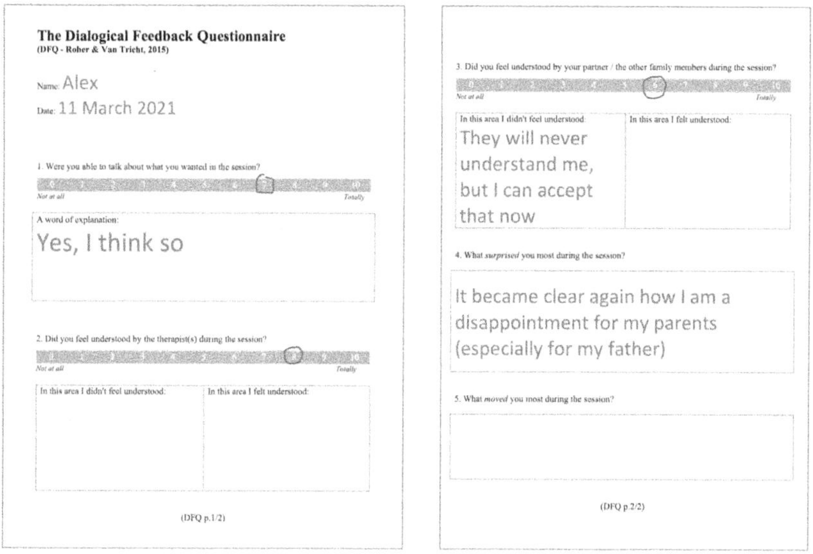

*Figure 7.1* Alex's DFQ (1st session).

I was surprised that Alex mentioned the disappointment of his parents (especially his father). I had seen sadness (mother) and irritation (father) in his parents, *but would they also be disappointed?* I thought of Alex as an only child, and of all the literature on only children that describe how only children are burdened by high parental expectations. *Is that what's going on here? Are the parents' expectations so high that Alex feels he can't live up to them? Does he try to meet them by setting himself sky-high goals, and then he can't help but fail ... ? Yes, maybe that could make the dynamics I observed in the family understandable.*

This is what father filled in on his DFQ:

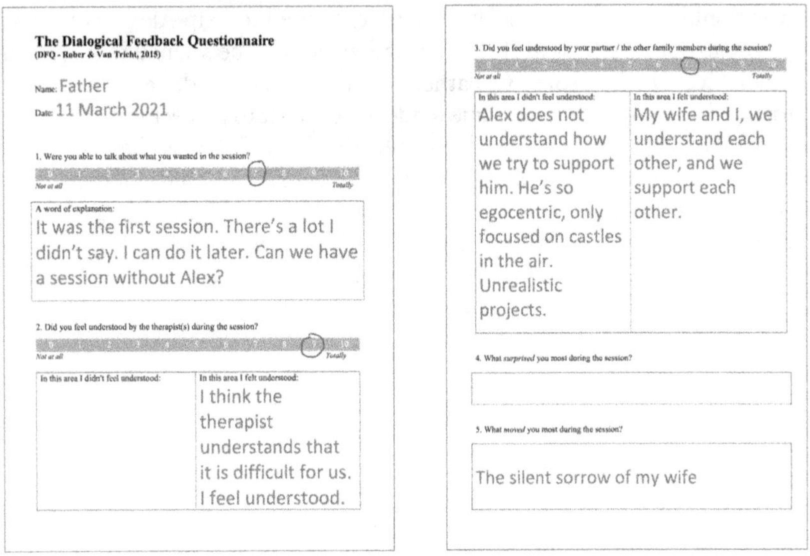

**The Dialogical Feedback Questionnaire**
(DFQ - Rober & Van Tricht, 2015)

Name: Father

Date: 11 March 2021

1. Were you able to talk about what you wanted in the session?

Not at all / Totally

A word of explanation:
It was the first session. There's a lot I didn't say. I can do it later. Can we have a session without Alex?

2. Did you feel understood by the therapist(s) during the session?

Not at all / Totally

| In this area I didn't feel understood: | In this area I felt understood: |
| --- | --- |
| | I think the therapist understands that it is difficult for us. I feel understood. |

3. Did you feel understood by your partner / the other family members during the session?

Not at all / Totally

| In this area I didn't feel understood: | In this area I felt understood: |
| --- | --- |
| Alex does not understand how we try to support him. He's so egocentric, only focused on castles in the air. Unrealistic projects. | My wife and I, we understand each other, and we support each other. |

4. What *surprised* you most during the session?

5. What *moved* you most during the session?

The silent sorrow of my wife

*Figure 7.2* Father's DFQ (1st session).

Father seemed to emphasize the bond with his wife. The support they find in each other. I also noticed that there was no irritation in his answers. Or at least much less than what I had felt in the session. Instead of irritation, there was concern and commitment. He writes "... that we do our best to support him". That is about his commitment and suffering: he wants to support Alex (commitment), but apparently, he feels that he is failing (suffering). I can work with that (irritation is much harder to work with). And then there was his request to speak with me, without Alex. Yes, maybe that wasn't a bad idea, if only because father would be able to express his irritation without pushing Alex even more into uncertainty and self-doubt. If father could talk to me about his irritation, and if I listened to him empathetically, he might feel heard and acknowledged, which would lessen his irritation, and that would benefit Alex. If … if … if.. There are still a lot of uncertainties, but now I have to make do with that.

This is the DFQ that mother filled in:

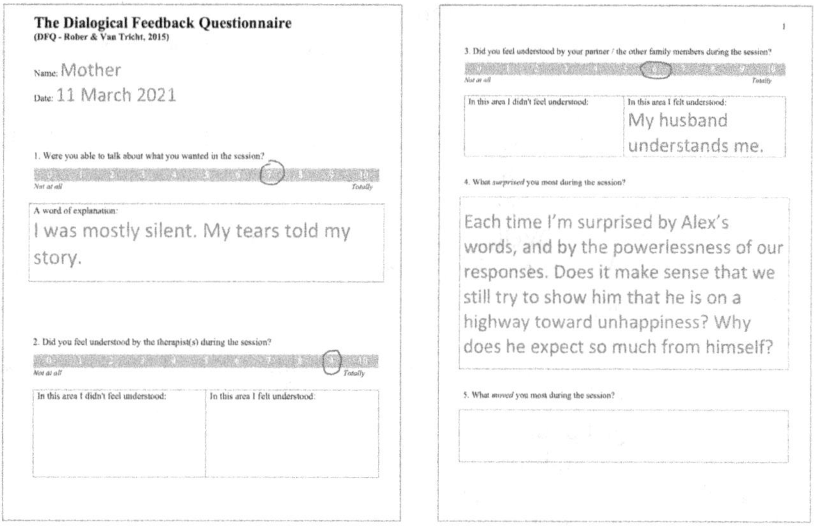

*Figure 7.3* Mother's DFQ (1st session).

As was already clear in the session, mother's sorrow is central to her, but her sorrow seems to be related to considerations that are very similar to father's considerations. She also emphasizes that she and her husband form a team together. They understand and support each other, although in the session he mainly expresses irritation, and she sadness.

*How can their answers to the feedback questionnaires help me in the next session?* I wondered. I might want to start (as I usually do) by returning their completed questionnaires to them and asking them if there's anything about in last session they want to talk about now.

### The second session

I gave each of them back their completed questionnaire, and asked, "Is there anything from the first session that you would like to come back to?"

They looked at the questionnaires and mother said, "Not really."

Alex shrugged.

Then father said, "I don't really want to go back on anything, but I'm curious what the others have written. Can we read each other's questionnaires? I'm especially curious about Alex's answers to the questions."

"That might be a good idea. At least if that feels comfortable for everyone ..."

Alex said, "It doesn't feel comfortable for me if they would read my questionnaire ..."

"That's fine, Alex," I said. "Is there a part of your questionnaire that feels ok to have read or maybe to read aloud?"

"Not really," Alex said. "They're going to be disappointed by what I've written."

"Be disappointed?" I asked.

Alex laughed for a moment. I think he realized what I also realized, which was that the theme of disappointment was so central to his answers to the questionnaire.

"Yes," Alex said. "Well, maybe I should read that piece ..."

Alex read aloud what he had written about being convinced that his parents were disappointed in him.

Father sighed.

Then Alex addressed his father and said: "Dad, I know I'm a disappointment to you ..."

Father shrugged and sighed.

I took the floor and turned to Alex.

"You feel like you're a disappointment to your father?" I asked, "Can you tell me a little bit more about that?"

"Yes, mmm, well, maybe every son is a disappointment to his father ... A baby is born and the first thing one asks is 'is it a boy or a girl?', and when you say it's a boy, they answer: 'congratulations, you will be very happy', and then as a father you are really happy of course. And then the child grows and with every small step you are proud of your son; the first laugh, the first word, the first steps ... But then the disappointment begins to seep in. And by the time the child is ten years old, as a father you must do your very best to hide your disappointment, and no matter how you try, your son starts to feel that he is falling short. It's starting to dawn on him that he's not living up to his father's expectations."

"That's how you experienced it?" I asked.

"No, no, that's the way it is with all sons, I think. Uh, well, so yes, consequently that's how I experienced it too."

I turned to father and asked him, "Do you think you were a disappointment to your father?"

I saw that my question surprised him. He might have expected me to continue to focus the conversation on his relationship with Alex, and now I suddenly addressed him as his father's son.

There was a moment of silence. *Understandable that he can't answer immediately*, I said to myself in my inner dialogue, *he has to switch gears.*

Father began to say, "Yes, I think I was a disappointment to my father. He was a doctor. A general practitioner. And I think he hoped and expected that I would become a doctor-specialist. But eventually I became a physiotherapist. He never said it openly, but I have always felt that a physiotherapist does not represent much in his eyes. Nothing really. He once told me, 'it doesn't matter what you become, as long as you become happy. And if being a physiotherapist is your dream, then that's ok for me'. I could taste the contempt for physiotherapy in his words."

"And becoming a physiotherapist was your dream?" I asked.

"No," Alex interrupted, "Dad actually wanted to be a professional cyclist."

That was surprising.

"Indeed," father continued, "I wanted to be a cyclist, but I didn't succeed. However, I had talent, and I really tried. At the age of 16 I started at the Lotto team as a youngster. In Belgium, the Lotto team is the big gateway to a professional contract. Everyone talked about my talent. And a few years later, I finished high school, and I had to choose what I would study at the university. Everybody said that it would be hard to combine studying medicine with my intensive training schedule as a pro cyclist. Physiotherapy would be less difficult to combine with cycling. So I decided to study physiotherapy. But eventually I had to stop cycling at the age of 20 when the team doctor based on my data started to suspect a slumbering heart disease. He sent me to a cardiologist and yes ... I had to say goodbye to my dream of a professional career as a cyclist."

"So you've disappointed your father by not becoming a doctor, and you've disappointed yourself by not becoming a pro cyclist," I said.

"And now I'm disappointing you because I don't care about the professional cycling," Alex added, "and because I want to be a writer."

"But no, Alex, *it doesn't matter what you become, as long as you become happy*," father said.

Alex was quick and wondered, tongue-in-cheek, "Where did I hear that phrase recently, dad? Oh yes, that's what Grandpa said to you ... "

Father fell silent and sighed.

It was quiet for a long time. Everyone was lost in thought.

"You're right Alex," father said softly.

"Am I right? That you echoed your father's words?"

"Yes, that too, but I meant, you're right that I'm disappointed in you. You always set your bar so high, over and over again, and of course you don't succeed, and then you're disappointed, and of course so am I."

Then mother jumped in: "And that hurts so much, Alex. As a parent, you mainly want your child to be happy, but we see you hit the same wall, each time again. Damn, don't you understand that we love you? Even if you're not an international celebrity or a champion?"

Until now I had only seen sadness in mother, but now I also saw anger. I also saw that Alex was shocked. To him, mother's anger was also surprising. And then I saw in the corner of my eye that father was groping for his handkerchief. He had tears in his eyes.

I spoke to father.

"What happens to you in the meantime?"

"Yes, my wife expresses it well. I also would like to see Alex carefree and happy. But he always puts himself under so much pressure."

"Yes," I said, "but in some ways you struggled with the same demons when you were growing up. How did you master your demons and then find a beautiful, sweet woman with whom you brought this beautiful son into the world ... How did you manage that?"

I saw Alex looking very interested, curious about what his father would say.

We talked more about ambition and disappointment, and about fathers and sons. At the end of the session, I asked them again to fill in the DFQ. While they were filling out the questionnaires, in my inner dialogue I was especially surprised by father, who had not been irritated at all during this session, and who had actually been very vulnerable. I was quite satisfied with the way the session had gone. I wondered how the family members had experienced the session.

Here's what Alex wrote:

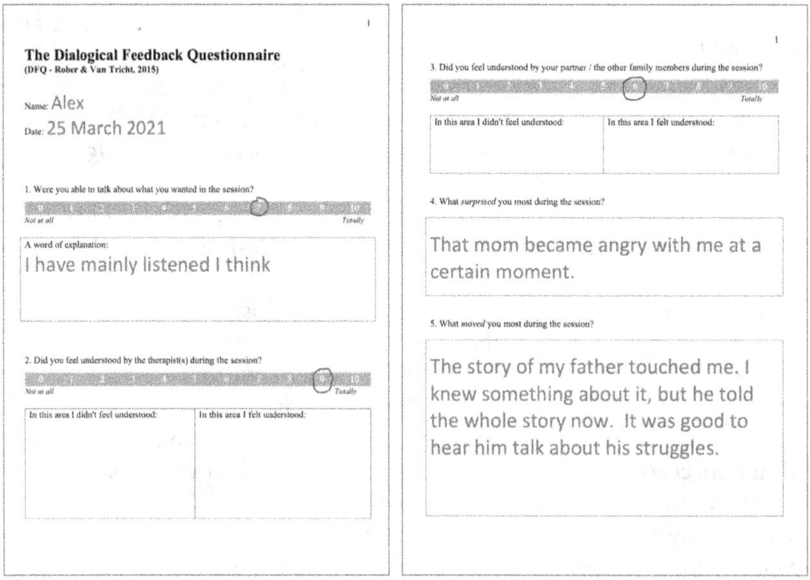

**The Dialogical Feedback Questionnaire**
(DFQ - Rober & Van Tricht, 2018)

Name: Alex

Date: 25 March 2021

1. Were you able to talk about what you wanted in the session?

Not at all — Totally

A word of explanation:
I have mainly listened I think

2. Did you feel understood by the therapist(s) during the session?

Not at all — Totally

In this area I didn't feel understood:       In this area I felt understood:

3. Did you feel understood by your partner / the other family members during the session?

Not at all — Totally

In this area I didn't feel understood:       In this area I felt understood:

4. What *surprised* you most during the session?

That mom became angry with me at a certain moment.

5. What *moved* you most during the session?

The story of my father touched me. I knew something about it, but he told the whole story now. It was good to hear him talk about his struggles.

*Figure 7.4* Alex's DFQ (2nd session).

When I read this, I felt confirmed in my impression that something new had happened between father and son. I was curious if that would also be reflected in father's DFQ.

This is father's DFQ:

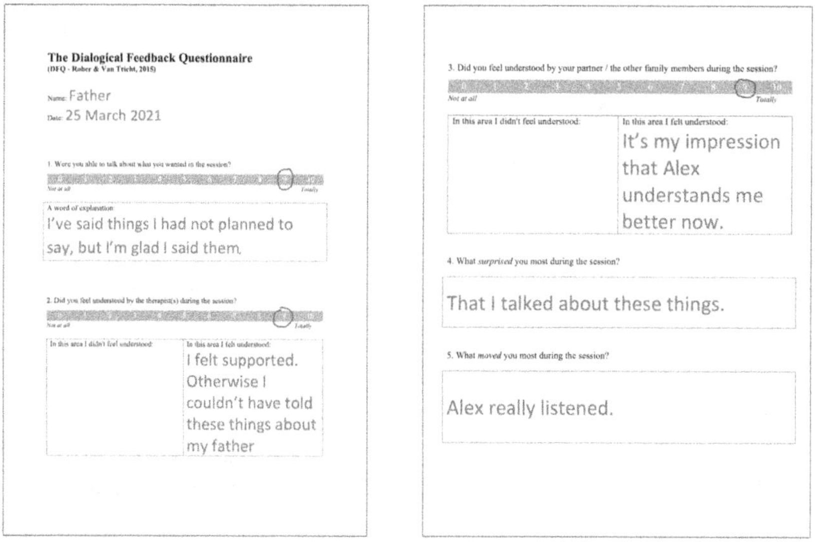

*Figure 7.5* Father's DFQ (2nd session).

Father's feedback suggests that something did indeed happen between him and his son in the session. It is also remarkable that he had surprised himself. He had said things that before the session he didn't think he would say. And – importantly – he didn't regret telling his son. He also felt how it seemed to have a good effect on Alex (" … that Alex understands me better now").

This is mother's DFQ:

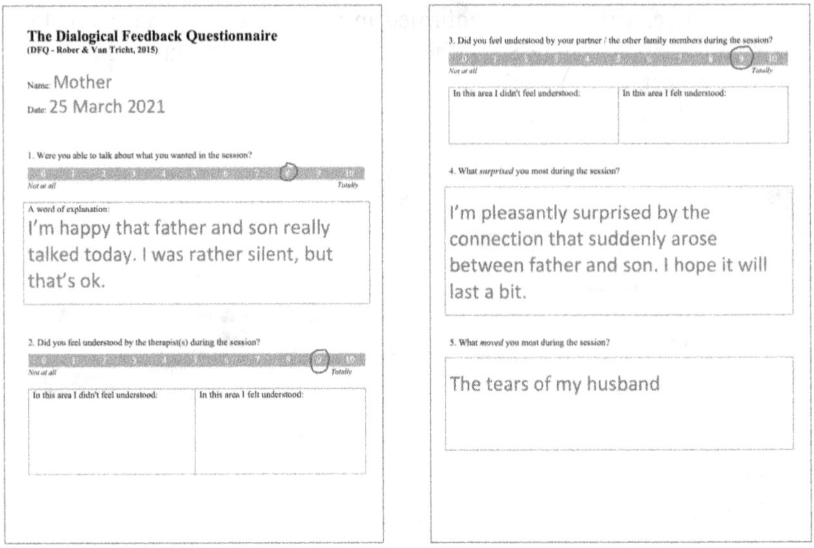

**The Dialogical Feedback Questionnaire**
(DFQ - Rober & Van Tricht, 2015)

Name: Mother
Date: 25 March 2021

1. Were you able to talk about what you wanted in the session?

*Not at all* — *Totally*

A word of explanation:
I'm happy that father and son really talked today. I was rather silent, but that's ok.

2. Did you feel understood by the therapist(s) during the session?

*Not at all* — *Totally*

| In this area I didn't feel understood: | In this area I felt understood: |
|---|---|
| | |

3. Did you feel understood by your partner / the other family members during the session?

*Not at all* — *Totally*

| In this area I didn't feel understood: | In this area I felt understood: |
|---|---|
| | |

4. What *surprised* you most during the session?

I'm pleasantly surprised by the connection that suddenly arose between father and son. I hope it will last a bit.

5. What *moved* you most during the session?

The tears of my husband

*Figure* 7.6 Mother's DFQ (2nd session).

When I read these answers, it dawned on me that in the 2nd session the parents had emotionally reversed roles. Mother had become angry, and father sad. I also liked that mother wrote that her husband's tears had touched her, where father had written after the first session that his wife's tears had touched him.

## Feedback tools as conversation tools

A feedback questionnaire such as the DFQ differs in several ways from other questionnaires used by family therapists as a feedback questionnaire. Some feedback questionnaires used by family therapists are in fact tools intended for individual therapy: for example, the SRS and the ORS (Duncan et al., 2003; Miller et al., 2003). There are also questionnaires that have been developed from a systemic perspective and can be used as a feedback tool, but were actually developed as research tools: for instance, the STIC (e.g. Pinsof, 2017) and the SCORE (Stratton et al., 2010). These are excellent instruments that have been extensively tested for their psychometric qualities (validity and reliability). An instrument like the Common Factors Feedback Interview (Karam & Blow, 2023) is very interesting for the use in families, but it is too long (15 open-ended questions) to use systematically at the end of every session.

The DFQ is different from most other feedback tools in a lot of respects. For one thing, while most feedback tools are meant to measure the effectiveness of the therapist and aim at collecting outcome feedback, the DFQ is focused on the therapeutic process. Its main goal is for the therapist to get a sense of how the different family members have experienced the session. Furthermore, the DFQ was not conceived as a measuring instrument. A measuring instrument is intended to obtain quantitative information about one or more variables. The psychometric properties of a measuring instrument can be calculated. The information generated by a measuring instrument can form the basis of graphic and software applications. The DFQ does not generate quantitative information as it was designed with a different objective, i.e. for use as a *conversational tool* (Sundet, 2014).

Questionnaires as conversational tools are not intended to give answers, but rather to raise interesting questions and topics to talk about in the session. For example, the answers provided by Alex and his parents on the DFQ sparked the therapist's inner dialogue. Their answers were not given a definitive interpretation but prompted the therapist's cautious reflections. Some of these reflections were used in the next session as a starting point for a dialogue with the family members. Used in this way, questionnaires as conversational tools can contribute to a better attunement between therapists and family members in terms of goals, themes, tempo, and so on. Such attunement is important because of its direct link with the quality of the therapeutic alliance.

## The purpose of feedback-oriented work

As the case of Alex and his parents demonstrates, feedback-oriented work in family therapy is more than collecting information. Rather, it is the starting point of self-reflection and dialogue. We refer here to the figure representing the three steps of feedback-oriented work.

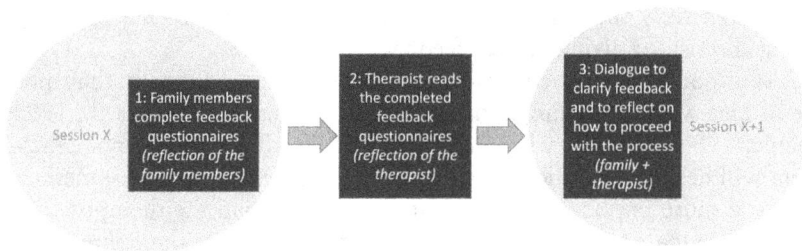

*Figure 7.7* Three steps in feedback-oriented work.

The process begins with the family members filling out the questionnaires (step 1). At that moment, they are invited to reflect on the way they have experienced the session. There is time for each family member to focus on his/her experiences and to find the words to express how they felt about the session. In step 2, the feedback from the family members will help the therapist to reflect on the therapeutic process in preparation for the next session. In addition, the feedback also invites the therapist to reflect about him/herself as a professional (professional self-doubt, see chapter 1), especially if some of the client feedback is of a critical nature. Finally, in step 3 the feedback-oriented work leads to dialogue between the therapist and the family members, but often also to dialogue between the family members.

### Client feedback is sometimes critical

Being feedback oriented as a therapist is primarily about making space for things that have not yet been said but may already be palpable in the conversation. This is well illustrated in the case of Alex and his family. The family members' feedback about the way they experienced the first session led me to reflect, and the discussion of the feedback questionnaires in the next session with a focus on a father's disappointment also made it possible for father to talk about the relationship with his father. This illustrates how a family member's feedback can be useful for the therapist to sharpen his/her curiosity and help him/her to find an orientation for the sessions that is better attuned to the family's own dynamics and history (Duncan, 2010).

What is not illustrated in the case of Alex and his parents is that client feedback can also be critical feedback towards the therapist. This can be challenging for the therapist because, when the client's feedback is critical, the therapist should be self-confident enough to not feel the need to justify him/herself or to explain what his/her good intentions have been in the previous session. He/she must instead channel his/her curiosity and try to better understand what the client is trying to say. The therapist should not react defensively, but rather he/she should be grateful to the client for taking the risk of giving critical feedback.

It is important that the therapist acknowledges the difficulty that most clients face when providing criticism of the therapist (e.g. Hill et al., 1993; Rennie, 1994). Usually, when completing the feedback questionnaire, the client will hesitate to criticize the therapist. This hesitation may sometimes lead to a more implicit or sugar-coated feedback, and the therapist must read the feedback carefully to pick up the criticism from the polite words written. Only if the client feels safe enough will he/she take the risk of openly giving critical feedback to the therapist (Rhodes et al., 1994). That is why it is important that the therapist invests in creating a culture of feedback (Prescott, 2017): a safe space in which the client can be sure that his/her feedback is welcome and will be taken seriously (Rober, 2017b).

Being open to the feedback of the clients makes the therapist vulnerable, and critical feedback is sometimes difficult to bear. The therapist then needs to regulate his/her own emotions (see Chapter 6) and must find a way to deal constructively with the client's criticism. This is illustrated in the next case with which will close this chapter.

### Stef, Isabel, and their father

I looked at the completed feedback questionnaires and I was disappointed. I even felt some anger. I had worked so hard to get them back in touch with each other and then after the session Stef had written on the questionnaire: "*is this all? Should we just accept what happened? Is it that simple: focus on the good moments with our father, and forget what happened? How disappointing.*"

I thought the session had gone well. Well, it had been a difficult session full of tension and I had found a way to bring the two adult children – Stef and Isabel – back into contact with their old father, despite their anger and disappointment. In the session with their father, the children had looked back on what had happened in their teens. A few years after the divorce of the parents – Isabel and Stef were 14 and 17 years old at the time – father had started a relationship with a new girlfriend, Els. He told his children that he expected them to accept Els. He also wanted them to understand that Els was not so patient and that she really wanted everything to go smoothly and quietly. She wanted the house tidy, and she couldn't stand it if the kitchen wasn't spick-and-span. But Isabel and Stef loved to stay in bed in the morning. They left bags of chips on the table near the TV when they went to bed late, because they would clean them up in the morning. So each time they were reprimanded by Els, and their father didn't stand up for them. He never took their side. On the contrary, he often took them aside to talk to them and make it clear that he expected them to behave and consider Els, who had to tolerate them.

"Remember," he would say, "she has chosen me, and because you are my children, she will take you. But she hasn't really chosen you yet."

"But dad, this is our house and she came to live here. And now she sets all the rules ..." Stef, the oldest, had said.

"No Stef," father had replied. "It's *my* house, and I want you both to make me proud and show Els that I raised you well."

After a few years, the relationship between father and Els ended. Father lived alone from then on. The children's relationship with their father improved, and Stef and Isabel grew up. They both went to college, they both fell in love, and they both started their own families. There were no more conflicts in the relationship between father and his children, and everyone seemed to enjoy the peace. But recently father fell in love again and started a relationship with An.

"There was a sudden outburst of distrust, and even anger and hostility," father said on the phone when he asked for an appointment. "I'm so happy with my relationship with An, but my kids don't want me to be in a relationship. It seems like they want me to stay alone for the rest of my life."

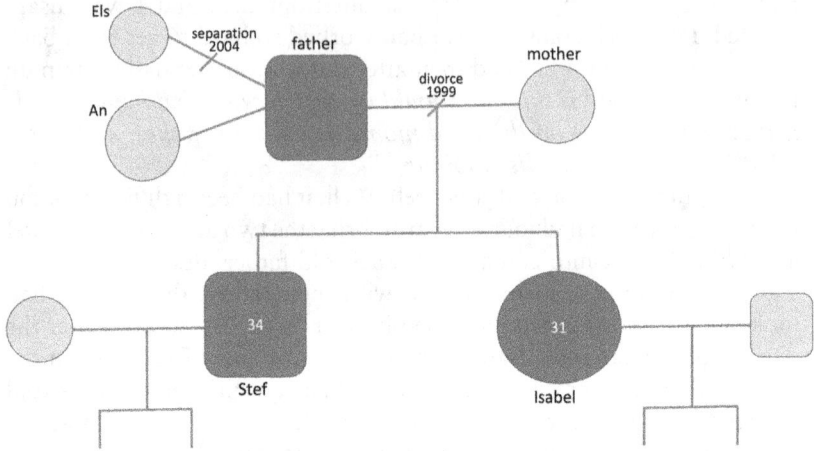

*Figure 7.8* Genogram Stef, Isabel and their family

In the first session, we talked about what had happened.

Stef was very clear in his opinions: "Dad, I'm glad you're happy now, but your relationship with An evokes so many bad memories of what happened in the years you were with Els."

"But that was almost 15 years ago. And you now have your own families. Partners. Children. You have your own home. And I have mine, and An lives with me now ..."

Stef said: "Yes, but then we will again come in second place for you. We will have to share you with An and you will always choose her side, no matter what we do."

"But you are adults now. 31 and 34 years old. You both have children of your own. Why should I put you first? I love both of you and your children, but I have my life and I love An too. We are a couple, and we are happy together. It is hard to stomach for me that you invite me to the birthday party of one of your children but An is not invited."

As a therapist, I sensed that I could understand father's point of view better than the children's. So I focused on Stef and Isabel, and I wanted to make an effort to understand them better.

"Stef and Isabel, it seems to me that what is happening now has nothing to do with the person of An?"

"Indeed, there is nothing wrong with An," Stef said, "She is a wonderful woman. We love her. But we don't want to lose our father and our children's grandfather. We don't want to experience the same thing as what happened to Els."

"Okay, what happened that you don't want to repeat?"

"We lost our father. He wasn't there for us," Isabel said.

"He let us down," Stef added.

"Did you talk to him about what that period really meant to both of you?"

"We tried," Isabel said, "but he doesn't understand. When we tried to talk about it in the past, he listened first and it felt good for a while, but then he wanted to explain that we didn't see it as it is, he would tell us how things really were, and he had excuses for everything that had happened."

"He doesn't see what it meant to us," Stef added. "I think he'll never understand because he's always so rational. When we are there with our emotions, we bump into his wall of his rationality."

Tense silence.

Then I said, "Well maybe you're right. Maybe your father is too rational. Perhaps there is an abyss between you and your father. Rationality versus emotions. I don't know. But if there is indeed the abyss, as you seem to suggest, then it may be something that cannot be changed. It's probably something your will have to accept." There was a brief silence. "But let's not be discouraged by the abyss, and let's look at the bridge that exists between the three of you. Tell me about the connection you have with each other. For example, tell me about the moments in the recent past when you really felt that you were there for each other."

The rest of the session we talked about the good moments between the children and their father. They were mainly moments when they could be alone with their father. Walks through the forest with dad. Together in the car on the way to the beach. The parties at home and the coziness by the fireplace. Talking about these moments created a nice and calm atmosphere in the session.

So, when I read the feedback questionnaires after the session, I was surprised and felt unfairly criticized by Stef. I had done my best to give something to each of the family members, and now it felt like I wasn't being recognized for my efforts. When I thought about the next session, I realized that my feeling of being criticized unjustly would be a bad starting point for the session.

I wondered if my disappointment and anger could maybe reflect something of what was happening in the family system. *Could my feelings help me get closer to what Stef and Isabel were feeling?* No, I didn't see how it fit. *But perhaps my feelings reflected something of what father had experienced.* Maybe. I knew I had to find a way to put aside my feelings of disappointment and anger or they would threaten the good alliance I had with them. I also realized that my anger was mainly directed at Stef and that I had to find a way to approach Stef authentically with empathy and curiosity despite my anger. At that moment, given the anger I felt, it seemed like an impossible task.

*Try to understand*, I told myself in my inner dialogue. *These three people love each other, and they had the best intentions. Still, things went wrong. And the result was disappointment and anger. You're the therapist, you have to try to understand that.*

This is how I started the second session.

After welcoming them, I asked, "How was the first session for you?"

Silence and hesitation. They looked at each other sheepishly and then studied the floor.

Then Stef broke the silence:

"Well, to be honest, I was disappointed. At one point it felt like you were saying to me 'accept it and move on with your life'."

"Can you help me understand your disappointment?" I said empathetically.

I had to put aside the explanations evoked in my inner dialogue about what I had tried to do in the first session and how my intentions had been good. I told myself to focus on Stef's words and try to understand him.

Stef explained how he experienced what had happened in the past as a grave injustice and that it was not possible for him to get over it.

Isabel said: "Yes, that's Stef. I'm different. This has happened so many times between Stef and me. He is my older brother and the knight who protected me. He always fights injustice. He wants to change things and that's fine. But some things can't change. The past, for example. You can't change that. What happened, happened. Focus on the future, Stef."

"Thanks, Isabel," I said, and I addressed Stef: "So, this is what happened the last session, Stef? You were disappointed because I wanted to focus on the moment of connection between you and your father, because it felt like I wanted to push aside the injustice in the past, that situation with Els?"

"Yes, it is," Stef said, "But I realize now that last time we didn't tell you what it was really about ... "

I was surprised, but I noticed that also Isabel looked at Stef incomprehensibly.

Father also didn't seem to understand what Stef was referring to.

"Yes," Stef said, "In fact, it wasn't primarily about dad's relationship with Els and how he neglected us. In fact, it was about what had happened in the years *before* his relationship with Els."

It was silent for a moment.

I was surprised by the turn the conversation took.

"So what had happened in the years before your father's relationship with Els?" I asked.

Stef told the story of the end of their parents' marriage, the four years before father met Els.

This is his story. When Stef was nine years old and his parents were still a couple, mother had a breakdown, because memories surfaced that she had been sexually abused by her father. This abuse began when the mother was nine years old and Stef's ninth birthday may have been the trigger for these memories to surface. Mother started to become psychologically unstable (depression, anxiety, etc.), and father tried to cope with that, but it did not work. Little Stef sensed something of what was happening and tried to support his mother as best he could. He stayed with her a lot and sometimes acted as if he was sick to stay home from school (he knew he could turn up the fever thermometer by quickly rubbing it with a handkerchief). He tried to cheer her up when she was down, and comfort her when she was sad. He also felt that things were not going well between father and mother. He feared that a divorce was imminent, and tried all he could to make both his parents happy in an attempt to keep them together. However, his efforts were not successful ...

After the divorce, the whole weight of his depressed mother fell on him.

"Then we felt completely let down," Stef said. "When dad left, I was 12 and Isabel was nine. We were left alone with our mother who was unpredictable, depressed, and anxious. Sometimes she was loving and took care of us, but sometimes she drank herself insensitive or had a panic attack. Sometimes she was happy, and then again depressed and when she was depressed, she sometimes talked about suicide. And we were supposed to be able to handle that ... I tried to help her as much as I could, but I couldn't."

"For me, the unpredictability was the most difficult," Isabel added. "Even if things were going well at home, it could suddenly turn into chaos, and we were powerless and alone. Where was dad?"

"Yes, the unpredictability was terrible," Stef said. "I always tried to be good, to be kind, to be perfect. That way, I hoped I wouldn't trigger her anger. And often it worked. I tried to be a good student at school, for example, getting good grades. That made my mother happy and proud. I kept my worries and sadness to myself so as not to evoke her disappointment because who knows, maybe she would drink too much again. So when she asked 'how was it today at school?' I always told beautiful stories about school, but I was alone with my grief when I had conflicts with my friends and or when I felt unfairly treated by the teacher. I had to bear my difficulties on my own."

I listened carefully to the story Stef and Isabel told me and it moved me deeply. I also have a past as a parentified child and although the circumstances were completely different, Stef's sense of responsibility and his powerlessness was something I could easily identify with. So when I empathetically said *what a heavy burden for two young children to bear* my words were marinated in my own history and I could feel a connection growing between me, Stef, and Isabel. I didn't have to explain anything about my own experiences in my family of origin. It was implicit in my presence in the room with them. They could tell that I understood what it means to be a child and feel like you have to take care of your mother who is struggling with issues beyond your comprehension and imagination.

"What a history you've had," I said. "And now I see you both sitting here in front of. Two beautiful young people. Both happily married and both loving parents of their own children. How did you manage to become such strong, independent adults with that difficult start you've had?"

Stef and Isabel were moved by my question.

They talked about their own families and how it had been challenging to start having children and how parenting is still some-times difficult.

"Especially when I get angry," Isabel said, "Then I need my husband to jump in. Over the years, he knows that. 'I'll take over here,' he says, and that gives me the opportunity to deal with my anger. I don't allow myself to be angry because it makes me feel guilty. Probably because it reminds me of the fear I had as a child when my mother got angry."

"For me, loving my children unconditionally is the most important thing," Stef said. "I want to be there for them so that they feel safe to come to me and talk about their worries and difficulties. I also want them not to have to worry about me. That they see that I am happy so that they can grow up unconcerned."

Silence.

At that moment I suddenly became aware that I had talked to Stef and Isabel the whole session so far. I looked at the clock, saw that it was almost time and father had not said anything yet. I had hardly given him any attention.

I turned to father and said:

"It's time to finish the session and I realize now that I didn't give you a chance to say anything. Sorry about that."

"That's ok," father said. "I've listened to them, and I've tried to understand."

"That's good," I said.

Silence.

I turned to father again and moved my chair just a little closer to his chair.

I leaned over to him and whispered, "You should be proud of your children."

Father tried to hold back his tears but then he started to cry.

He couldn't speak but he tried to say he's proud. The words sounded strange, but we all understood what he meant.

Isabel got up and sat down with her father. She hugged him tightly.

We ended the session in silence.

I asked them to fill out the feedback questionnaires.

Father wrote, "I have never been so proud of my children".

Isabel's feedback: "warm feeling. I feel close to dad".

Stef's feedback: "good session. Father listened and seemed to understand. For the first time".

# 8 The Self-Supervision Questionnaire[1]

In this chapter, I propose a tool that can help family therapists reflect on the families they work with, and more specifically on the complex alliance they have with families.

The Self-Supervision Questionnaire (SSQ) (see attachment 3) is structured similarly to the Dialogical Feedback Questionnaire (DFQ) (see chapter 7) and consists of five questions. The focus is on the experience of the therapist and on the relationship of the therapist with the different family members.

It is a questionnaire that helps me reflect on my role as a therapist, and on my own experience of the session. For instance, question 3 invites reflection on the discomfort of the therapist, which I talked about in chapter 6. I fill out this questionnaire at the end of the session while the family members are filling out their feedback questionnaires. Before the start of the next session, I will then review the completed feedback questionnaires and the SSQ to prepare for the session.

I have noticed that the SSQ adds something substantial to the notes I routinely make during the session and to what I recall about the session. On the one hand, my answers to the questions bring me closer to the way I actually experienced the session, and on the other hand, these answers when I read them offer me a perspective from a certain distance and that helps me to think about the process of the therapy. In that way, the SSQ is a very useful addition to the feedback questionnaires that the clients have completed when preparing for a family therapy session.

In the discussion of the following case, I will not pay a lot of attention to the feedback questionnaires completed by the family. Instead, my focus will be on the use of the Self-Supervision Questionnaire.

---

1 Download for free via https://www.intherapytogether.com/.

DOI: 10.4324/9781003458395-14

## Lyka and her family

Lyka is 18 years old. She and her family have been referred for family therapy by the psychiatrist at a hospital that specializes in treating young people with eating disorders. She had been hospitalized for about two months and she was doing better now. However, the psychiatrist wanted there to be some kind of follow-up for Lyka and also for the family.

In the first session the whole family was present: Lyka, her older brother Daan (21 years old), and their parents. Each of them had completed the Worries Questionnaire (see chapter 2) in advance. From their answers I understood that all were motivated for the therapy. That's why it was surprising that in the session, while we were getting acquainted, they were all so silent. They gave friendly but brief answers to my open-ended questions. *A quiet family*, I noted in my inner dialogue. I also noticed that the parents were very careful in the way they talked to Lyka.

I mentioned this, and mother said:

"We're so relieved that she recovered from her eating disorder."

"What do you mean?" I asked. I didn't see how their relief was connected with the silences and the way in which they measured their talk so carefully.

"We wouldn't want her to start fasting and throwing up again."

"You're afraid you'd say something wrong?"

"Yes."

Father added: "It's strange to realize that we spent years trying to help her, but no matter what we tried, it only got worse. Only when she was in the hospital, she started to get better."

"Mmm," I said, but I wasn't sure I understood what he meant. I let father's words sink in. Several questions bubbled up in my inner dialogue. *Did he mean that they felt it was their fault that she had developed an eating disorder in the first place? Or did he mean that they hadn't handled it well as parents, and that now they were afraid to say something wrong that might lead to a re-awakening of the eating disorder?*

"Are you afraid to say something wrong that could cause her to relapse?" I asked.

"Yes."

"Oh, so by being quiet you take care of each other?" I spoke.

"Yes," father said, "sometimes silence is best."

Then it was quiet again, but the silence somehow felt different. I had the impression that my words brought relief to the parents. At the time, I didn't make much of it, but in hindsight, maybe I should have sensed that there was a family secret at play.

At the end of the session, everyone filled out the feedback questionnaire (DFQ). I completed the Self-Supervision Questionnaire.

As I prepared for the next session with Lyka's family, I looked at the feedback questionnaires the family members had filled out. I was particularly struck by the fact that everybody felt understood. I also noticed that all the family members were very hopeful. *It was a good first session, and we're on the right track*, seemed to be the main message. I also looked at the SSQ that I had filled out myself.

This is the questionnaire as I filled it out after the first session:

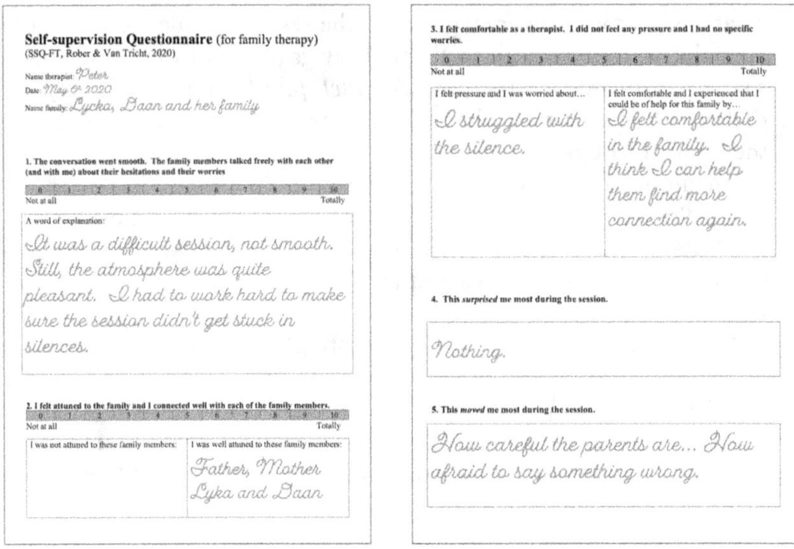

**Self-supervision Questionnaire** (for family therapy)
(SSQ-FT, Rober & Van Tricht, 2020)

Name therapist: Peter
Date: May 6th 2020
Name family: Lycka, Daan and her family

**1. The conversation went smooth. The family members talked freely with each other (and with me) about their hesitations and their worries**

| 0 | 1 | 2 | 3 | 4 | 5 | 6 | 7 | 8 | 9 | 10 |
|---|---|---|---|---|---|---|---|---|---|---|

Not at all — Totally

A word of explanation:
It was a difficult session, not smooth. Still, the atmosphere was quite pleasant. I had to work hard to make sure the session didn't get stuck in silences.

**2. I felt attuned to the family and I connected well with each of the family members.**

| 0 | 1 | 2 | 3 | 4 | 5 | 6 | 7 | 8 | 9 | 10 |
|---|---|---|---|---|---|---|---|---|---|---|

Not at all — Totally

| I was not attuned to these family members: | I was well attuned to these family members: |
|---|---|
| | Father, Mother Lyka and Daan |

**3. I felt comfortable as a therapist. I did not feel any pressure and I had no specific worries.**

| 0 | 1 | 2 | 3 | 4 | 5 | 6 | 7 | 8 | 9 | 10 |
|---|---|---|---|---|---|---|---|---|---|---|

Not at all — Totally

| I felt pressure and I was worried about… | I felt comfortable and I experienced that I could be of help for this family by… |
|---|---|
| I struggled with the silence. | I felt comfortable in the family. I think I can help them find more connection again. |

**4. This *surprised* me most during the session.**

Nothing.

**5. This *moved* me most during the session.**

How careful the parents are… How afraid to say something wrong.

*Figure 8.1* My Self-Supervision Questionnaire after the 1st session.

I noticed how I had struggled with the silences in the family. It was actually exhausting as a therapist to search for openings all the time and to deal constructively with those silences. In fact, maybe it was remarkable that I had not been irritated. *Fortunately*, I reflected, *I like them. Otherwise, the long silences and their thoughtful way of talking might begin to annoy me.*

I realized that I had to do something with the silences in the session to avoid jeopardizing our good relationship due to my impending irritation. The best way I knew of dealing with this was to try to share something with the family about my experiences. But how could I share my thoughts about the exhausting silences with the family without them feeling criticized? I sensed their vulnerability, and I wanted to avoid them feeling accused. On the other hand, I myself should avoid being silenced about the silence that was so pervasive in the session. I looked at the SSQ again. Yes, in answer to question 3 I had written that I struggled with the silences. I have learned that it is often important to do something constructive with what I have written about in terms of discomfort. That's often the challenge: How to talk about your discomfort as a therapist, in such a way that it is helpful for the family? In a way that it opens space in the session to talk about difficult issues that were unspoken until then? Another thing that struck me was my answer to the 4th question (about what had surprised me the most in the session). I had written "nothing". This worried me, because the answer to that question often says something about the usefulness of the therapy. It is my experience that in sessions where I am more surprised (question 4), or more moved by things (question 5), that there also is more warm connection in the family. If *nothing* surprises me in the session, this often indicates an impasse or a therapy that is stuck. *Have I become too cautious with them*, I wondered. *Is the silence in the family contagious? Do I want to protect them from their difficult feelings and their painful experiences? Maybe I'm like the parents who are afraid to speak and say things that can stir up emotions in Lyka? Or maybe I'm taking care of my own comfort by avoiding difficult themes? Have I snuggled too much into my comfort out of sympathy for this family? Maybe I have to take more risks in the next session? I have to try to get some emotional depth in the session, but I think that also means that I have to become more vulnerable myself.* These are some of the thoughts that floated in my inner dialogue while I was preparing for the session.

I started the session with the general question "how are you?". I didn't address anyone in particular.

A long silence followed. When rewatching the video recording of the session, I measured the duration of the silence: 18 seconds.

I broke the silence and said:

"That's a big silence."

More silence (seven seconds).

"Are there any thoughts about the previous session?" I tried.

At that moment, weird electronic sounds suddenly broke the silence. Daan was startled and reached for his iPhone in his backpack.

"Sorry," he said, "I'll turn it off."

"Cool ringtone," I said.

"Yes, it's the intro to a Stromae song," Daan replied.

"Really?" I said. "What song?"

"It's called *Silence*. It's on his *Cheese* album."

"Silence? How appropriate … just when we were starting to drown in silence …" I said jokingly.

Everyone laughed.

"You are champions of silence," I continued addressing no one in particular. "How did you become so good at silences?"

Silence (five seconds).

Then Daan said:

"Sometimes I don't know what to say."

"You don't know what to say?"

"Yes, well, I usually know what to say, but I don't know if it would be a good idea to speak."

"What do you keep quiet about the most? About the things that are too unimportant to talk about, or about the things that are so important that it's hard to talk about them?"

Daan thought for a moment (silence of four seconds) and then he said: "I wouldn't want to hurt anyone. That's often why I'm silent."

"And are you more concerned about *their* vulnerability than your *own?*"

"I'm more concerned about them," Daan said, glancing at Lyka.

"So talking here in the session is difficult for you, Daan?"

"Yes."

"I think you're in good company," I said jokingly.

I looked at the other family members.

"You're all very good at silences, aren't you?"

Everyone nodded.

"It's not that you are not involved in the session, but you are very careful in what you share with the others. Right?"

Everyone nodded, but it remained silent (four seconds).

Lyka then said: "As Daan said, we don't want to hurt each other, but for me, I also feel vulnerable and afraid of being hurt if I share things that are very personal."

"Mmm," I said.

Silence (three seconds).

Mom said: "Sometimes it's like my words make the others silent. That's why I don't say much."

"Mmm," I said.

Silence (three seconds).

*Hey,* I noticed that dad's eyes were getting moist. *What is going on?* Only then did I realize that he hadn't said anything in the whole session.

I asked, "And dad, how's it for you?"

He said: "I also think sometimes the kids are silent because they don't want us to worry. Children often take care of their parents."

A few tears rolled down his cheeks. In a way, I was happy to see these tears. It meant that an emotional connection with the family was growing and that they felt safe enough with me to show their vulnerability. And it also meant that they felt safe enough together to share these emotions with each other. I looked around to see how the others reacted to father's tears. I saw mother offering paper tissues to her husband. Both Daan and Lyka now had tears in their eyes. The silence was filled with emotion and a sense of togetherness. While I didn't understand exactly where father's tears came from, I let it happen without asking any further questions. Only in the next session would I be able to see the connection between the theme of silence and father's tears.

At the end of the session, the family members completed the feedback questionnaires. I filled out the SSQ.

Here's what I replied to the questions:

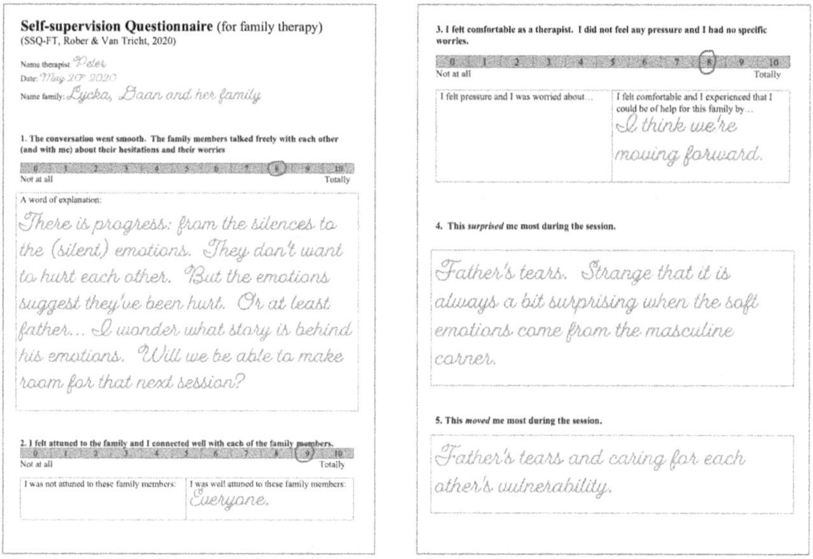

**Self-supervision Questionnaire** (for family therapy)
(SSQ-FT, Rober & Van Tricht, 2020)

Name therapist: Peter
Date: May 20th 2020
Name family: Lycka, Daan and her family

**1. The conversation went smooth. The family members talked freely with each other (and with me) about their hesitations and their worries**

0 1 2 3 4 5 6 7 (8) 9 10
Not at all ... Totally

A word of explanation:
There is progress: from the silences to the (silent) emotions. They don't want to hurt each other. But the emotions suggest they've been hurt. Or at least father... I wonder what story is behind his emotions. Will we be able to make room for that next session?

**2. I felt attuned to the family and I connected well with each of the family members.**

0 1 2 3 4 5 6 7 8 (9) 10
Not at all ... Totally

| I was not attuned to these family members: | I was well attuned to these family members: |
|---|---|
| | Everyone. |

**3. I felt comfortable as a therapist. I did not feel any pressure and I had no specific worries.**

0 1 2 3 4 5 6 7 (8) 9 10
Not at all ... Totally

| I felt pressure and I was worried about… | I felt comfortable and I experienced that I could be of help for this family by… |
|---|---|
| | I think we're moving forward. |

**4. This *surprised* me most during the session.**

Father's tears. Strange that it is always a bit surprising when the soft emotions come from the masculine corner.

**5. This *moved* me most during the session.**

Father's tears and caring for each other's vulnerability.

*Figure 8.2* My Self-Supervision Questionnaire after the 2nd session.

Two weeks later both the feedback questionnaires and the SSQ proved to be useful to prepare for the next session. From the feedback questionnaires, I learned that they all thought it was a good session. They felt understood by me (average 9/10), and also by each other (average 9/10). Both Lyka and Daan went on to write that they were touched by father's tears. Mother wrote that she was surprised that her husband had showed his emotions: "I haven't seen him like this very often", she wrote.

The answers to their feedback questionnaires seemed to confirm quite a bit what I already sensed. I took a careful look at the SSQ and thought that I had captured the session well with my answer to the first question: there was progress in the sense that emotions and a sense of togetherness came into the session, but the emotions remained silent and not connected to a story. In retrospect, I realised I hadn't even tried to ask father to tell the story of his tears. The thought of asking him hadn't even crossed my mind in the session. *Why? Was I focused on my own comfort again? Or was I reluctant because the emotions came "from the masculine corner", as I wrote in my answer to question 4? I'm not afraid of my emotions myself (I think), but maybe I wanted to protect father by avoiding the story of his emotions? That would fit nicely with the family dynamic: taking care of each other's vulnerability by avoiding talking. Yes, maybe I was infected by the family's virus?* I resolved to continue working in the next session as in the first sessions (because I noticed that there was progress in the therapeutic relationship), but also to try to make room for father's story of his tears.

I started the next session by giving the completed feedback questionnaires from the previous session to the family members, asking "is there anything from previous session that you want to come back to?".

A long silence (20 seconds) followed.

Then I said to father, "Last session I was quite surprised by your tears, and I noticed afterwards that I didn't ask you to explain where your tears came from."

Father seemed quite startled by my question.

"It was a moment of weakness," he said.

"Or a moment of strength, in which you had the courage to show how you felt?" I tried.

Silence (four seconds).

"That's not easy for us men," I continued.

I didn't know what to ask, but I wanted to take risks carefully, so I joined the themes that had bubbled up in my reflections on last session. By referring to "us men" I also tried to strengthen my bond with him.

Mother addressed her husband: "You don't usually do that ... you never show your emotions."

Silence (7 seconds).

Then I asked father: "What example did your father give you about how to deal with emotions as a man?"

Silence (6 seconds), but I saw tears coming back into father's eyes.

My question evoked a lot, but I didn't understand what exactly.

"My father died early ..." father said softly.

He made no eye contact and looked at the floor. As if he was embarrassed. *Something important is happening here* flashed through my mind, *but I still don't understand.*

Daan took the floor: "He had cancer and died when daddy was six years old."

*He's taking care of his dad* flashed through my inner dialogue, but my thoughts were abruptly cut short by father: "No, he didn't die of cancer, son. He committed suicide."

As if a bomb exploded. The children looked at their father with wide eyes.

Eyes of disbelief.

Silence (two seconds).

Mother broke the silence and addressed me:

"We never told the kids. His father committed suicide when he was six, but we told the children that he died of cancer."

Silence (four seconds).

Father said, "We wanted to protect them, and they were still so young. How were we supposed to explain what suicide is? We wanted to tell them later, when the children were a little older and when they would understand it better. But we never talked about it."

Silence (14 seconds).

I turned to father: "I understand," I said. "Yes, it is difficult to explain to children what suicide is. But you yourself were only six when your father died. How did you understand it then?"

"Yes, I was six. I knew he had committed suicide. I don't remember exactly how I knew, but I knew. Later, my father's death was never talked about. I was an only child, so I was left with my mother. I've always thought she felt guilty about his suicide. But I'm not sure. She became depressed. That colored pretty much my childhood. I had to take care of my mother. I wanted to keep her from getting depressed. The most important thing was to be quiet and remain silent."

Silence (four seconds).

"Can you give an example?" I asked.

"Well, after my father's death, my mother wanted me to sleep with her every night. She didn't dare sleep alone. So, I slept with her every night. But she had nightmares, and she would cry in her sleep. I could tell from her crying and moaning that that she dreamed about my father. She tossed and turned and cried and wept. I lay awake beside her. But in the morning when we got up and she asked, 'did you sleep well?' I always said that I had slept very well. I didn't want to alarm her."

The rest of the session we talked about father's childhood, the next sessions too, and it became obvious how silence had become both their protection and their prison. The evolution of the therapy was positive: there was gradually more connection in the family and after 12 sessions we stopped the therapy.

# *Stairway to heaven:* Jason Sonck and his family (part 3)

"You're the worst therapist in the world," Jason had said before slamming the door.

The therapy with the Sonck family then stopped. Jason didn't want to come back.

After the session in which Jason walked away, I had one more session with the parents. But the session didn't really come to life. Perhaps also because of my insecurity and self-doubt. Yes, Jason's words had left traces. Father suggested not to make a new appointment for the time being.

Months later I received an email from Jason's father. He informed me that Jason was still struggling, but that there was a turnaround:

**Dear Peter,**

Jason is in love. It's like the sun breaking through the clouds. Yes, there are still many clouds because his mood swings and temper tantrums remain difficult to bear, especially for his mother but also for me. But now that he has met Marie, we sometimes see him happy. Marie is a girl he met in the self-help group for traffic victims with a brain injury. She also was in an accident – hit by a bus – which mainly left her with headaches, cognitive impairment, and language disorders.

Marie is a sweet girl. We first met her last week when Jason brought her home for dinner. It was nice to see him happy again. In such moments he shows that he is happy to be alive again. Although the next day it was the same again. He had a temper tantrum in his room and smashed a guitar (which he regretted afterwards).

Anyway, I wanted to let you know that there are still dark clouds, but there are also clearances.

DOI: 10.4324/9781003458395-15

> Thanks for the sessions, Peter. I often think back of them. The therapy has been an important support for us, and it still is.
> Best regards
> Joris Sonck (Jason's dad)

I sent back a short message: "Thanks for the weather forecast. I'm glad there are more clearances and that you now and then see that Jason is happy to live."

I didn't hear from the Sonck family for a long time.

Three years later, I received a birth announcement: "Jimmy is born. The parents Marie and Jason are very proud of their dear son."

I sent them a card with congratulations. I also sent a short note to Jason's mother and father to congratulate them on their grandparenting.

I got a long email back from father, with a few pictures of Jimmy, Marie, and Jason. Father wrote that the young family was doing well and that Jason was no longer talking about euthanasia: "He has a sense of life again and he loves Jimmy dearly. I think he's already making plans to teach Jimmy to play the guitar."

# Part IV
# Being a family therapist

# 9 The story of the therapy with the De Smet family

## The first session

The De Smet family arrived right on time for their first session. The application form read: "Parents are worried about their daughter Fran (22 years old) injuring herself. She cuts her arms. She's also depressed."

Before I met the family, I looked at the Worries Questionnaires they filled out (see chapter 2). From this I could conclude that both parents were very worried, and that Fran herself was rather hesitant. Yes, she knew her parents were worried about her, but she wasn't that worried herself. She went on to write that she wasn't sure what to expect from family therapy: "at least I don't really see how therapy might be useful for us". So I immediately got a clue about the dynamic I could expect in the first session: the parents were the *doorkeepers* who took the initiative, and Fran was the window-shopping *visitor* (see Chapter 2).

In the session I met father and mother with their two daughters: Fran and Jacoba (20 years old).

When I asked them who had referred them, father surprisingly said: "Jason Sonck." (See the narrative intermezzos, part 1–3.)

I was confused for a moment as the name Jason Sonck rang a bell, I couldn't place him very well. Then I thought back to the jerky and stuttering young man who wanted to die, and to his parents who wanted to keep him alive. I thought back to Jason's ambitions to be as good a guitar player as Jimmy Page, and to his pain and sadness because he would never be able to perform the complex solo of *Stairway To Heaven* on stage again.

"Jason Sonck? The guitar player?" I asked.

"Yes," said father, "I used to attend workshops on rock guitar with him. Yes, I also play guitar myself. Even after his accident he still is a good guitar player, and he is an excellent teacher. A few months ago, I met him by chance at a rock concert in Brussels, and we went for a pint together after the concert. I had then told him something about

DOI: 10.4324/9781003458395-17

our concerns about Fran, and how hard it was on the family. Jason then said, 'Go talk to Peter Rober. He is the best therapist in Belgium.'"

I couldn't suppress a smile.

Then I asked the family members to introduce themselves. Father began. He is a social worker at a health insurance fund, and in his spare time he plays lead guitar in an amateur band that plays *Status Quo* covers. Mother is a social worker for the social services of the city of Brussels. She also does quite a bit of sports: jogging and walking (which they often do together as a family). Jacoba studies nursing and is a volunteer at the animal shelter where she cleans animal cages and goes for walks with dogs. Fran hesitated before she said anything about herself. Then she said that she recently graduated as a biologist and that she is now at home. She is not yet sure what kind of job she wants to have. In fact, she had started studying biology because she was fascinated by the figure of Jane Goodall, the well-known primatologist. Fran was surprised that I knew who Jane Goodall was, and that I could refer to a *National Geographic* documentary about her. Fran then told me that she would have liked to work with bonobos. That could possibly be in the animal park Plankendael, where they have a large community of bonobos, but there had not been any job opportunities for biologists for a long time, so now she did not know what she wanted to do as a biologist.

After this introduction, the parents said that Fran had been isolating herself for a long time in the family. She retired to her room and only came down during meals. The parents were worried about her, even though they didn't know at first that Fran was cutting herself. They only discovered this later after mother found a bloodied handkerchief in the laundry basket. Fran had cut too deep and had tried to stem the blood with the help of that handkerchief.

I looked at Fran for a moment: a young woman, somewhat set, and with Buddy Holly glasses on her nose. Rather classically dressed. I immediately noticed the big difference with her sister, who was much slimmer. Short hair and boyishly dressed, yet very feminine and fresh. Jacoba somehow felt to me like much more open than Fran. Yes, it was not easy for me to connect with Fran. It felt like she kept me at a distance. On the one hand, I respected that, but I also wanted her to feel that I wanted to be there for her. I did feel that she appreciated that I knew who Jane Goodall was. But otherwise, she was rather reluctant, which is to be expected from a visitor. I was aware that this caused the same thing to happen in the session with me as with the parents at home: just as she had been keeping her parents at a distance for months, she also kept me at bay.

I looked at Jacoba and wondered what role she played in the family dynamics. Jacoba seemed to understand very well how difficult it was for her parents that Fran kept them at a distance. She herself had more contact with her sister: sometimes they went to the gym together and then they talked a bit. But since Fran had gone to Leuven to study, there had been a distance between them. Now Fran had graduated, and she was living back home. However, the distance between the two sisters hardly diminished. In the session I saw that Jacoba mediated between the parents and Fran. When the parents said something to Fran and Fran did not answer immediately, Jacoba sometimes rephrased what her parents had said in her own words. And vice versa: a few times it happened that Jacoba picked up something that Fran had said and explained it further to her parents and me under the approving eye of her sister.

This gave me a first insight into the dynamics in the family: the parents were very worried and were looking for a connection with Fran. Fran was struggling with her own things and kept her parents at a distance. Jacoba tried to be a bridge. I described this after the session in the Self Supervision Questionnaire (see chapter 8). I went on to write, "I didn't really manage to tune in to Fran, despite my honest attempts (I didn't want to scare her away either)". I also wrote that what touched me the most was the gap between the parents and Fran.

### The next sessions (sessions 2–5)

In the following sessions, there gradually was somewhat more trust in the family. In the beginning Fran was very hesitant about therapy, but she slowly came loose in the next sessions. She began to talk more about her fears and insecurities. "Am I good enough?" was the question she often asked herself. For instance, this question arose when she thought of her 2 best friends who – in her opinion – were much more beautiful. "Maybe I'm not good enough to be friends with them", she wondered. She also asked herself that question when she fell in love with a boy, and when that boy invited her on a date: "Am I good enough for him?" She could not go to her parents with these questions. Yes, they would listen to her, but they wouldn't understand it, Fran told herself. I wondered in my inner dialogue, *doesn't Fran trust them? Or doesn't she allow herself to rely on her parents as a young adult?* I didn't know. Anyway, Fran imagined that her parents were never insecure and never doubted themselves. And then she looked at herself in the mirror, and she would see someone who was failing and someone who was scared witless. Cutting herself brought peace at such moments.

For the parents, it was a relief to finally hear their daughter talk about what she was going through. However, it was also painful because in the sessions it appeared that Fran had felt lonely all these years and that she had kept her parents at a distance because she was convinced that her parents would not understand her. From that conviction also grew the anger towards her parents that sporadically reared its head. And then fierce conflicts arose in which the parents tried to make their good intentions clear, in which Fran accused them of not understanding anything at all. Jacoba mediated between the conflicting parties.

At times Fran was able to talk a little more openly about her doubts in the sessions, and that gave the parents the opportunity to assure her that she could always come to them.

"We will always be there for you," mother said with tears in her eyes.

Fran's cold reaction, however, showed that she didn't know if she could believe her mother's words. Jacoba tried to be a bridge as always, but that didn't really work out well because Fran also started to keep her at a distance.

The sessions with Fran and her family remained difficult. *At least they are sitting together and trying to connect*, I wrote on the SSQ after the fifth session. I noticed that in the sessions I gradually started to take on the role of Jacoba: like her, I also tried to be a bridge between Fran and her parents. I sensed that they loved each other, and that they needed each other, but somehow, they didn't find the connection. On the one hand, I saw Fran, who was afraid of the big outside world and felt insecure. On the other hand, I saw the parents trying to support their daughter and trying to give her advice. They didn't see that their advice wasn't helpful to Fran, who understood the advice as a lack of confidence in her.

"You tell me how to go about it," Fran said at one point, "because you don't trust me to do it well myself."

In that way, the good intentions of the parents collided with Fran's fears and insecurities.

There was something else. Fran had always been the good student and she was also the first and only in the family to obtain a master's degree at the university. Also, in high school she had always been the best, certainly in comparison with Jacoba for whom school had always been more difficult. In the fifth session, Fran said that she had started to experience all this as a pressure: she had to be an example for her sister and always perform well.

"It has cost me an awful lot and it exhausted me," Fran said. "I always had to be perfect, but I'm not perfect."

She said she started keeping her parents at a distance because she thought her parents would be disappointed in her if they saw who she really was and that she wasn't as perfect as she made it out to be. Here, too, the important question played a role for her: "Am I good enough?"

When Fran told all this in the fifth session, this seemed like a big leap forward. But the feedback questionnaires (see chapter 7) after the session taught me that I was too optimistic. All four family members felt discouraged in their answers to the questions about how they had experienced the session. Mother wrote that it was painful to notice that her daughter was keeping her at a distance. Father wrote: "I try to support my wife because it hurts her a lot that Fran doesn't trust her. It hurts me too". Jacoba wrote: "we are running around in circles. We've been around about five times already, and we can't find a way out".

This feedback made me fully realize that the therapy had stalled. Jacoba was right, I had tried the same thing over and over again because I thought I saw opportunities for the parents and the daughter to find each other, but when it didn't work out, I encouraged myself and just tried again. Now that I took the time to sort it out, I could only conclude that it would never work out this way. That took my breath away and I thought: *If I can't get Fran and her parents to connect with each other, what should I do then?* I looked at the feedback questionnaires again and then Fran's feedback struck me: "their sermons don't help me", she wrote, "my parents don't know how hard it is for me. I cannot blame them for not understanding. How can adults understand how difficult it is to grow up?". This feedback surprised me and got me thinking. For Fran, the most important thing seemed to be that she didn't feel understood. Her question suddenly seemed very relevant to me: "how can adults understand how difficult it is to grow up?".

I resolved to ask the parents in the next session to talk about their own growing up. *How did they themselves grow up? How did they gain confidence when they started to break free from home?* This seemed like an interesting new angle: inviting the parents to talk about the stage of life Fran was struggling with now. Asking them to talk about their childhood and their first steps into adulthood. Perhaps that would also help them to have a better understanding of the difficulties Fran is struggling with. And maybe it would help Fran to believe in the possibility that her parents would understand her. I did not know what the effect of this change of course would be, but I felt hopeful again and was excited to continue working with this family.

### The sixth session

I asked both parents to talk about their own growing up:
"How did you as 20–22-year-olds find your way to independence?"
I suggested Fran and Jacoba just listen, and then I addressed the parents: "Who is going to start?"

Mother said she always was a good daughter. Working well for school, going to music class to learn to play the piano, helping in the household, etc.

"I had a younger brother Dirk. He was a rebel. He was always different and didn't shy away from conflict. He didn't want to go to music class, and he didn't want to go to the boy scouts. He had few friends, and he often kept his distance. Actually, I never knew him well. He had his own life. My parents worried a lot about him, and that pushed me even more to be good so as not to make them worry about me. Then I went to study in Antwerp, and that's where I met my husband, Daan. I was already 20 at the time. Daan took me by the hand, as it were, and he sweetly led me away from my parents. Actually, it has been very soft and gradual. For him–" (she nodded her head in the direction of father)– "growing up has been much more painful."

She looked at her husband, inviting him to tell his story.

Father said that he also studied as a social worker, but that he was actually more interested in music: "I played guitar in a rock band and that was my passion. I felt that I didn't have the talent to really be a professional musician, but I still took music very seriously. Everyone in our band did, by the way. Music was our life. Not only the music we played but also the music we listened to. My father was not interested in music. He even made a bit of a mockery of it. When I was listening to a CD with my headphones, he would tap me on the shoulder so that I would take off my headphones and then he would ask if I was torturing my ears again with what he called 'loud noise'. Music really didn't interest him. In fact, that hurt me, but I didn't tell anyone, especially not him."

"Especially not him?" I asked.

"No, I mainly wanted to show him that I didn't need him. I wanted to prove that I could stand on my own two feet."

I looked at Fran and saw that she was listening intently. She looked at her sister for a moment and then back at father. In my inner dialogue (see chapter 5), I thought: *maybe she listens so carefully because there are similarities between her parents' stories and hers. Mother who tried to be the perfect daughter, for example, and father who kept his distance from his parents in an attempt to prove himself.*

Father went on to say:

"The only thing my father considered important were my grades in school. He had not been able to study himself due to circumstances (his family was really poor), and he has always carried that with him as a lifelong setback. It meant a lot to him that I would continue on after high school to become a social worker. I think he was proud of me, but he never said it."

"He never said it?"

"No, he never said it. Not then and not later because he died before I graduated. A heart attack."

I noticed tears in father's eyes.

I was curious if the other family members had noticed it too.

Mother took over: "I already knew Daan at that time. We were both living in student's apartments in Antwerp."

This gave father the chance to take a handkerchief and dry his tears.

"Yes," mother continued. "It happened so suddenly. One day he was still there, and then suddenly there was a phone call from Daan's mother to say that his father had died."

"I've never been able to talk it out with him," father said, "I still regret that a lot. And it sometimes weighs on my relationship with Fran. I'm so afraid that she would suddenly be gone, and that she wouldn't realize how much we love her despite everything."

Now I saw tears in Fran's eyes.

Her sister gave her the box of Kleenex.

It was silent for a long time in the session. A sense of belonging lingered and it was as if everyone allowed themselves to taste it for a while.

I let the silence last, and I was curious who would break it.

That turned out to be Fran. She addressed her parents.

"We didn't know that," Fran said, "you never told us."

I noticed that she said "we" and "us". Until now, she had always talked about "I" and had always presented herself as a misunderstood and insecure loner. And now she put herself side by side with her sister.

"Yes," Jacoba added. "It's nice to hear this."

The session was coming to an end. I suggested to Fran and Jacoba that they prepare an interview with their parents together for the next session.

"What questions do you have about your parents' childhood? And about the period that they got to know each other and decided to form a family together. We'll make time for the interview next time."

The feedback questionnaires taught me that everyone had experienced this session as very useful. Mother wrote that she was touched by the way the children had listened: "quiet and present". Fran wrote that her father's story had touched her: "I've never seen my father like that before".

In retrospect, this sixth session was very important. At the end of the therapy, Fran told me that this session was a turning point for her. After this session, she hadn't cut herself anymore.

### The seventh session

The interview was well prepared by the girls and their parents talked with much emotion about their childhood and their fledgling relationship. Fran asked her parents what had attracted them to each other, and she also wanted to know how they had decided to get married. I noticed that Fran in particular asked the questions and talked to her parents, while Jacoba was rather quiet. Actually, Jacoba only asked a few questions about mother's younger brother, Dirk. "Uncle Dirk", the girls called him. They didn't know him well, because he lived in Paris. They had only seen him a few times at parties.

Fran said: "We don't know much about Uncle Dirk."

Jacoba added: "We only know he's *a fag*. He is effeminate."

What struck me were not so much her words, but rather the way she spoke them. No, it did not sound negative, nor reproachful, on the contrary. She seemed fascinated by her uncle.

Jacoba's fascination with her gay uncle came back to mind when I read in the feedback questionnaire that she wanted to talk about her *gender* in the next session. "I've wanted to talk about it for a long time", she wrote, "but my sister and her problems were always central. Rightly. Now that Fran is doing better, maybe next time we can talk about my struggle with being a woman".

### Eighth session

At the beginning of the session, I suggested that, following up on what Jacoba had written on her feedback questionnaire, attention should be paid to the things she was struggling with.

The fact that Jacoba was struggling with her womanhood was new to me, but no one in the family seemed surprised. Jacoba thought that no one had noticed, but actually everyone knew that she was struggling with herself, with her body and with her sexuality.

So when she said, "I have to tell you something, and I hope you're not going to let me down," father, mother, and Fran already had a strong suspicion of what it would be about.

Then Jacoba said that for years she sometimes fell in love with a boy and then again with a girl. She also felt that she was actually a boy, and that her body was wrong. She said she hadn't felt well in her woman's body for many years. She had struggled with herself in silence, wondering who she really was. She hadn't talked to anyone about it.

No one was surprised and above all there was relief when Jacoba brought this up in the session. Father and mother asked some questions, and Jacoba mainly said that she had no answers. Jacoba seemed relieved because she felt that the reactions of her parents and her sister were supportive, without a trace of reproach or negative connotations

"You seem relieved, Jacoba?" I asked.

"Yes, I really feel supported by mom and dad, and also by my sister. I was so afraid that they would reject me. I am grateful to them."

She cried. Fran moved her chair closer and put her hand on Jacoba's shoulder.

Silence.

Jacoba then told me that she had been on a quest for a long time to find out who she really was. She said that she had found a lot of websites and blogs where she read about gender dysphoria, transgenderism, sexual identity, and so on.

"It has strengthened my belief that I am in the wrong body," Jacoba said.

Everyone nodded and smiled.

There was an atmosphere of connectedness in the session.

"And now," Jacoba continued, "I'm ready for the next step. I went to Ghent, to the gender team at the academic hospital, to make an appointment for treatment."

Father responded curiously: "Treatment?"

"Yes, there is a center for sexology and gender there," Jacoba said, "and when I went there, I had a consultation with a doctor who is specialized in transgenderism. I have opted for a gender-affirming treatment."

Fran asked: "A gender-affirming treatment? What's that?"

"It is a process from caterpillar to butterfly. You come out of your cocoon, as it were, so that you can really be who you are."

"Nice, but that sounds like a sales pitch," said father. "How exactly does such a treatment go?"

There was a moment of silence. As if Jacoba had to find the courage to continue.

"The first thing that's going to happen is that they're going to take away my breasts," Jacoba said.

I was shocked. Somehow I hadn't expected this.

The others also seemed shocked. On father's face I could read his bewilderment.

It was very quiet in the session.

A deep silence, which mother finally broke.

"We knew that you were struggling with your gender, Jacoba," said mother, "but that you would immediately opt for a major operation … "

"It's not 'immediately', I've been thinking about it for years. I've read a lot about it and talked to people who know something about it. People who are trans themselves. And then I went to Ghent. I spoke to the specialists there, and now my decision is final."

Silence.

I decided to try to be a bridge between Jacoba and her parents.

"For you, this decision is not sudden, Jacoba. You prepared it well. But for your parents, it is sudden. They didn't expect it," I said.

"I had feared this," Jacoba said, "but I had hoped that my parents would want me to be happy."

"We want you to be happy," father tried. "But have you thought about this enough?"

We talked a bit more about the steps Jacoba wanted to take but it was clear that nothing more could be said in this session that would bring the parents and Jacoba closer together. I handed out the feedback questionnaires and we made a new appointment.

### My reflections after the eighth session

I looked at the completed feedback questionnaires (see chapter 7) and Jacoba's especially stood out. She wrote that she had not felt understood by me (4/10) and that I had been on the side of father, mother, and Fran. That surprised me. I looked at the Self Supervision Questionnaire that I had completed after the session. I found in it that in my feeling I was equally attuned to everyone. To the third question of the questionnaire, I did answer that I was worried about Jacoba's choice. "So drastic and irreversible", I wrote, and also, "if it were my daughter, I would be very worried". I noticed now that I had clearly taken the perspective of a father here. I thought about it further, and I was reminded of Jason Sonck. Remarkable that he came to mind. In Jason's case it was not at all about transgenderism. But I did see a similarity. In both cases it was about choices of young people that are irreversible: Jason wanted to die, and Jacoba wanted to have her breasts removed. I had learned from my experiences with Jason that sometimes it's good not to make such a radical choice, because things can happen in your life that make it all look different later on. He wanted to die, but now he is happy that he is alive and that he can pass on life to his son. What if Jacoba has her breasts cut away and regrets it afterwards?

Those thoughts went through my head as I thought about Jacoba's decision to have surgery, and I felt what it did to me. I know myself and I know that I am not at all negative about transgenderism. I thought I had been open and understanding to Jacoba in the session, as I had been to each of the family members. But that clearly wasn't Jacoba's sense. I tried to check with myself what had been going on with me. I remember looking at Jacoba, at her face which was indeed boyish, and at her body which had undeniably a feminine shape. Her clothes couldn't hide it. And then the idea that she would have her breasts cut away ... "if it was my daughter ..." Yes, the realization began to dawn on me that I had listened with the ears of the parents.

I resolved to try to get out of the position of the parents next session, and really listen to Jacoba. I could do that by coming less to the foreground myself and by giving the parents more space. If they took on more of their parenting role in the session, it would be easier for me not to do it. I realized that it was also true the other way around: if I did not take on the parent role in the session, it would be easier for them to do so.

### The ninth session

I started the session with the question:
"Is there anything from the previous session that you want to talk about?"
Silence.
Then I said that I had been very affected by Jacoba's feedback questionnaire. I said: "Thank you, Jacoba for what you have written."
When I heard myself say it, I thought it sounded sincere, and Jacoba's reaction seemed to point in the same direction.
So I continued: "I've been thinking about it a lot in the preparation of this session, and I realize you're right. It was certainly not my intention, and I was not aware of it at the time, but I now see that I was looking at you through the eyes of a father. And I now realize that I left you out in the cold. I'm terribly sorry about that. I'm going to try not to do that anymore. But keep giving me feedback if I don't succeed."
It was quiet for a moment and then Jacoba said: "Thanks."
Long silence.
Then father said: "Can I also say something about last time? I've felt guilty after last session. Not about my reaction to what Jacoba said, but rather because 20 years ago, when Jacoba was born, I was disappointed that she was not a boy. We already had a daughter and I really wanted to have a son this time. During the pregnancy I only fantasized about a son. We even had a name for a son: Jacob, and we didn't even consider a maiden name. And then there was the birth, and then it turned out to be a daughter. I couldn't believe it at first, and we hadn't come up with a name for a girl. That's why we called her Jacoba. Yes, I struggled with it for months, but gradually that went away. I thought Jacoba was a fantastic baby. And after a while I was happy that I had 2 daughters. I really enjoyed watching them grow up together."
"Mmm, but you talked about feeling guilty," I said. "So where is your guilt then?"
"Well, I think Jacoba might have felt when she was little that I initially wanted a son. Maybe that's why she has such a hard time accepting her womanhood."
Jacoba had listened carefully and after a while she shook her head.

"No, that has nothing to do with it, Dad. I didn't even know," she said. It was silent for a moment.

Then mother started to speak.

"I'm sorry you don't want to be a woman," mother said. "And it also evokes something of guilt in me: haven't I taught you enough how beautiful it is to be a woman?"

Throughout the session, the four family members exchanged views. They did not agree, but they could each give their vision and they listened to each other. There were emotions and tears. No one was left untouched. As a therapist, I was able to stay out of the discussion. I could sympathize with each of them. That was also evident from the feedback questionnaires that the family members filled in afterwards. Everyone felt understood by me (all scores of 8 and 9 on the second question).

The conclusion of the session was that mother, father, and Fran regretted that Jacoba opted for such a radical treatment, and that Jacoba stood by her decision. But before we ended the session, Fran had another comment.

She said, "Sister, listen. If you need surgery like that to be happy, I'm all for it. I've known for a long time that you feel like half a boy. What I have a particularly hard time with, Jacoba, is that you want to have your breasts cut away. After all, we went to therapy because I cut myself. And now that I don't do that anymore, you want to cut yourself ... " She turned to me. "Isn't this also a kind of self-mutilation ... 'non-suicidal self-injury'?"

Everyone was looking at me. They seemed to expect an answer, but I didn't know what to say.

So Jacoba took the floor: "It's a medical procedure, it's not a disease."

"Yes, "said Fran, "but it's much more drastic than the cutting I did. My wounds healed by themselves, but what you want to do is irreversible."

Silence.

"I also think it's weird," Fran continued. "You have such a beautiful body. I've always been jealous of your body. And you have beautiful breasts. And you want to get rid of them, Jacoba?"

"Yes, I want to get rid of them because they make me feel uncomfortable. I can't be myself in a woman's body. I've made my mind up. Jacoba is a thing of the past. From now on I'm Jacob."

### Finally

The therapy continued for several months. Jacoba is now Jacob, and it is actually no longer a point of discussion in the family.

# Epilogue

Family therapy can be conceptualized in many different ways, and this book was written against the background of a conceptualization of family therapy as a dialogue of living persons (Rober, 2005a). Such a conceptualization offers a perspective that makes it possible to capture something of the mutuality and shared activity of a therapeutic encounter in practice.

It could be argued, of course, that the expression 'a dialogue of living persons' is a tautology, given that all persons in dialogue are living – how else could they interact or communicate? Emphasizing these persons' vitality, however, directs our attention, not to their behavior nor to the content of these persons' stories, but rather to the existential fact that these persons are all breathing, their hearts are beating, and they have concerns, dreams, disappointments, memories, and fears. These persons are alive, and they are also relational beings, because they are involved with their surroundings, continuously tuned in to each other and interacting with each other. Yes, the concept of family therapy as a dialogical meeting of living persons can help us to think and talk about the relational and responsively created nature of a family therapy session.

Within such a conceptualization, the therapist is an active, responsive listener. Moving back and forth between positions of identification and of outsideness, he/she tries to understand the different family members and is focused on making room for the multiplicity of voices of the family. The therapist is not only interested in sameness, but also in difference, as he/she is open to unexpected meanings that emerge in the session. These meanings may threaten the brittle equilibrium in the family, or they can throw a new light on things so that novel ways of living together become possible.

If we describe family therapy as a dialogical meeting of living persons, this is what we see happening in the session: The family members are strongly connected, although that may be far from obvious as what dominates their interactions may be disappointment, fear, and anger. Still, they are oriented towards each other: one speaks, another responds.

Sometimes they agree, but often they don't. There are invitations, negotiations, and coordinated dances. There are words and silences filled with what is left unspoken. There is time and it is irreversible – a ceaseless flow of moments, all unique, all sacred, in which we are immersed. There is wonder and fear, beauty and uncertainty, good intentions and remorse, boredom and surprise. There is pain and love, and everything in between.

And the therapist must be able to endure powerlessness. There will always be more suffering than a therapist can heal. Even a perfect therapist would fall short. And there is no such thing as a perfect therapist. We therapists are committed to try to alleviate psychological suffering and we do it as best we can. We are not perfect, and that is acceptable if we are focused on learning and becoming more effective.

And whatever happens, the therapist is present; listening to each family member, sensing their suffering, realistically believing in them, seeing hope in the love between them that is there somewhere, but often hidden because of the disappointment and pain ...

This is how frail a dialogue of living persons is.

This is how full of potential it is.

# References

Abramson, M. & Goldinger, S.D. (1997). What the reader's eye tells the mind's ear: Silent reading activates inner speech. *Perception and Psychophysics, 59,* 1059–1068.

Alderson-Day, B. & Fernyhough, C. (2015). Inner Speech: Development, cognitive functions, phenomenology, and Neurobiology. *Psychological Bulletin, 141,* 931–965.

Allen, P., Aleman, A., & McGuire, P.K. (2007). Inner Speech Models of Auditory Verbal Hallucinations: Evidence from behavioural and neuroimaging studies. *International Review of Psychiatry, 19*(4), 407–415.

Amble, I., Gude, T., Stubdal, S., Andersen, B.J., & Wampold, B.E. (2015). The effect of implementing the Outcome Questionnaire-45.2 feedback system in Norway: A multisite randomized clinical trial in a naturalistic setting. *Psychotherapy Research, 25,* 669–677.

Anderson, H. & Goolishian, H. (1992). The Client Is The Expert: a Not-Knowing Approach to Therapy. In McNamee, S. & Gergen, K.J. (Eds.). *Therapy as Social Construction* (pp. 25–39). London: Sage.

Anderson, T., Ogles, B.M., Patterson, C.L., Lambert, M.J., & Vermeersch, D.A. (2009). Therapist Effects: Facilitative interpersonal skills as predictors of therapist success. *Journal of Clinical Psychology, 65,* 755–768.

Anderson, T. & Hill, C.E. (2017). The role of therapist skills in therapist effectiveness. In Castonguay, L.G. & Hill, C.E. (Eds.). *How and why are some therapists better than other? Understanding therapist effects* (pp. 139–158). Washington, DC: American Psychological Association.

Andolfi, M., Angelo, C., & de Nichilo, M. (1989). *The Myth of Atlas: Families & The Therapeutic Story.* New York: Brunner/Mazel.

Andolfi, M. (1995). The Child as Consultant. In: Andolfi, M. & Haber, R. (Eds.). *Please help me with this family* (pp. 73–89). New York: Brunner/Mazel.

Anker, M. G., Duncan, B. L., & Sparks, J. A. (2009). Using client feedback to improve couple therapy outcomes: A randomized clinical trial in a naturalistic setting. *Journal of Consulting and Clinical Psychology, 77*(4), 693–704.

Aponte, H.J. & Carlsen, J.C. (2009). An instrument for person-of-the-therapist supervision. *Journal of Marital and Family Therapy, 35,* 395–405.

Aponte, H.J., & Kissil, K. (2014). 'If I can grapple with this I can truly be of use in the therapy room': Using the therapist's own emotional struggles to facilitate effective therapy. *Journal of Marital and Family Therapy, 40,* 152–164.

Aponte, H.J. & Kissil, K. (Eds.) (2016). *The Person of the Therapist Training Model: Mastering the use of self* (pp. 94–108). New York: Routledge.

Arnold, M. B. (1960). *Emotion and personality.* New York: Columbia University Press.

Bachelor, A., & Horvath, A. (1999). The therapeutic relationship. In Hubble, M.A., Duncan, B.L. & Miller, S.D. (Eds.). *The heart and soul of change: What works in therapy* (pp. 133–178). Washington, DC: APA Press.

Bakhtin, M. (1981). *The dialogic imagination.* Austin, TX: University of Texas Press.

Bakhtin, M. (1984). *Problems of Dostoevsky's poetics.* Minneapolis: University of Minneapolis Press.

Bakhtin, M. (1986). *Speech genres & other late essays.* Austin, TX: University of Texas Press.

Baldwin, S.A. & Imel, Z.E. (2013). Therapist Effects: Findings and methods. In M.J. Lambert (Ed.). *Bergin & Garfield's Handbook of Psychotherapy and Behavior Change* (6th edition, pp. 258–297), New York: Wiley.

Barkham, M., Lutz, W., Lambert, M.J., & Saxon, D. (2017). Therapist effects, effective therapists and the law of variability. In Castonguay, L.G. & Hill, C.E. (Eds.). *How and why are some therapists better than others? Understanding therapist effects* (pp. 13–36). Washington, DC: American Psychological Association.

Barkham, M. & Lambert, M.J. (2021). The efficacy and effectiveness of psychological therapies. In Barkham, M., Lutz, W., & Castonguay, L.G. (Eds.). *Bergin and Garfield's Handbook of Psychotherapy and Behavior Change* (pp. 135–189). Hoboken, NJ: Wiley.

Barkham, M., De Jong, K., Delgadillo, J., & Lutz, W. (2023). Routine Outcome Monitoring (ROM) and Feedback: Research review and recommendations. *Psychotherapy Research, 33,* 7, 841–855.

Bateman, A. & Fonagy, P. (2004). *Psychotherapy for Borderline Personality Disorder: Mentalization Based Treatment.* Oxford: Oxford University Press.

Bateson, G. (1979). *Mind and Nature: A necessary Unity.* New York: E.P. Dutton.

Bermudez, J.L. (2018). Inner Speech Determinacy and thinking consciously about thoughts. In Langland-Hassan, P. & Vicente, A. (Eds.). *Inner Speech: New Voices* (pp. 199–220). Oxford, UK: Oxford University Press.

Bertrando, P. & Gilli, G. (2010). Theories of change and the practice of systemic supervision. In Burck, C. & Daniel, G. (Eds.). *Mirrors and reflections: Processes of systemic supervision* (pp. 3–26). London: Karnac.

Beutler, L.E., Malik, M., Alimohamed, S., Harwood, T.M., Talebi, H., & Noble, S. (2004). Therapist variables. In Lambert, M.J. (Ed.). *Bergin & Garfield's Handbook of Psychotherapy and Behavior Change* (5th edition, pp. 227–306), New York: Wiley.

Beutler, L.E., Bongar, B., & Shurkin, J.N. (1998). *A consumer's guide to psychotherapy.* New York: Oxford University Press.

Blow, A.J., Seedall, R.B., Miller, D.L., Rousmaniere, T., & Vaz, A. (2023). *Deliberate Practice in Systemic Family Therapy*. Washington, DC: American Psychological Association.

Bohart, A.C. & Greaves Wade, A. (2013). The client in psychotherapy. In Lambert, M.J. (Ed.). *Bergin & Garfield's Handbook of Psychotherapy and Behavior Change* (6th edition, pp. 219–257), New York: Wiley.

Boss, P.G. (1987). The role of intuition in family research: Three issues of ethics. *Contemporary Family Therapy*, 9, 146–159. doi:10.1007/BF00890270

Boszormenyi-Nagy, I. & Spark, G. (1973). *Invisible loyalties: Reciprocity in intergenerational family therapy*. New York: Harper & Row.

Bowen, M. (1972). Toward a differentiation of a self in one's family. In Framo, J.L. (Ed.). *Family interaction* (pp. 111–173). New York: Springer.

Bowlby J. (1969). *Attachment and Loss. Vol.1: Attachment*. New York: Basic Books.

Bowlby, J. (1988). *A Secure Base: Parent-Child attachment and healthy human development*. New York: Basic Books.

Bruner, J. S. (1973). *The relevance of education*. New York: Norton.

Bruner, J.S. (2004). The narrative creation of self. In Angus, L.E. & McLeod, J. (Eds.). *The Handbook of Narrative and Psychotherapy: Practice, theory and research* (pp. 3–14). London: Sage.

Buber, M. (1923,2013). *I and thou*. London: Bloomsbury.

Byng-Hall, J. (1995). *Rewriting Family Scripts: Improvisation and Systems Change*. New York: Guilford.

Carruthers, P. (2018). The Causes and Contents of Inner Speech. In Langland-Hassan, P. & Vicente, A. (Eds.). *Inner Speech: New Voices* (pp. 31–52). Oxford, UK: Oxford University Press.

Castonguay, L.G. & Hill, C.E. (Eds.) (2017). *How and why are some therapists better than other? Understanding therapist effects*. Washington, DC: American Psychological Association.

Chow, D.L. (2014). *The Study of Supershrinks: Development and deliberate practice of highly effective psychotherapists* (unpublished doctoral dissertation). Perth, Australia: Curtin University.

Chow, D.L. (2017). The Practice and the Practical: Pushing your clinical performance to the next level. In Prescott, D.S., Maeschalck, C.L., & Miller, S.D. (Eds.). *Feedback Informed Treatment in Clinical Practice: Reaching for excellence* (p.323–355). Washington, D.C.: American Psychological Association.

Clark, A. (2019). *Surfing Uncertainty: Prediction, action and the embodied mind*. New York: Oxford University Press.

Constantino, M.J., Vîslă, A., Coyne, A.E., & Boswell, J.F. (2019). Cultivating Positive Outcome Expectations. In Norcross, J.C. & Lambert, M.J. (Eds.). *Psychotherapy Relationships That Work: Vol.1 Evidence-Based Therapist Contributions* (pp. 461–494). New York: Oxford University Press.

Crits-Christoph, P. & Connolly Gibbons, M.B. (2021). Psychotherapy Process-Outcome Research: Advances in Understanding Causal Connections. In Barkham, M., Lutz, W., & Castonguay, L.G. (Eds.). *Bergin and Garfield's*

*Handbook of Psychotherapy and Behavior Change* (pp. 263–295). Hoboken, NJ: Wiley.

Dalenberg, C.J. (2004). Maintaining the safe and effective therapeutic relationship in the context of distrust and anger. *Psychotherapy, 41*, 438–447.

Damasio, A.R. (1994). *Descartes' Error*. New York: G.P. Putnam's Sons.

Dawes, R.M. (1994). *House of cards: Psychology and psychotherapy built on myth*. New York: Free Press.

Dozier, M. & Tyrrell, C. (1998). The role of attachment in therapeutic relationships. In Simons, J.A. & Rholes, W.S. (Eds.). *Attachment theory and close relationships* (pp. 221–248). New York: Guilford Press.

de Jong, K., van Sluis, P., Nutger, M.A., Heiser, W.J. & Spinhoven, P. (2014). Understanding the differential impact of outcome monitoring: Therapist variables that moderate feedback effects in a randomized clinical trial. *Psychotherapy Research, 22*, 464–474.

De Shazer, S. (1988). *Clues: Investigating solutions in brief therapy*. New York: Norton.

Dijksterhuis, A., Bos, M.W., Nordgren, L.F., & van Baaren, R.B. (2006). On making the right choice: the deliberation-without-attention effect. *Science, 311*, 1005–1007.

Duncan, B.L. (2010). *On becoming a better therapist*. Washington, DC: American Psychological Association.

Duncan, B.L. & Miller, S.D. (2000). *The heroic client: Doing client-directed, outcome-informed therapy*. New York: John Wiley.

Duncan, B.L., Miller, S.D., Sparks, J.A., Claud, D.A., Reynolds, L.R., Brown, J., & Johnson, L.D. (2003). The Session Rating Scale: Preliminary Psychometric Properties of a "Working" Alliance Measure. *Journal of Brief Therapy, 3*, 3–12.

Elkaïm, M. (1997). *If you love me, don't love me: Undoing reciprocal double binds and other methods of change in marital and family therapy*. Northvale, NJ: Jason Aronson.

Elliott, R., Bohart, A.C., Watson, J.C., & Murphy, D. (2019). Empathy. In Norcross, J.C. & Lambert, M.J. (Eds.). *Psychotherapy Relationships That Work: Vol.1 Evidence-Based Therapist Contributions* (pp. 245–287). New York: Oxford University Press.

Engel, P.J.H. (2008). Tacit knowledge and visual expertise in medical diagnostic reasoning: Implications for medical education. *Medical Teacher, 30*, e184–e188.

Escudero, V & Friedlander, M.J. (2017). *Therapeutic Alliances with Families: Empowering clients in challenging cases*. Cham, Switzerland: Springer.

Evans, J.St.B.T. (2003). In two minds: Dual process accounts of reasoning. *Trends in Cognitive Sciences, 7*(10), 454–459.

Evans, J.St.B.T. (2008). Dual processing accounts of reasoning, judgment, and social cognition. *Annual Review of Psychology, 59*, 255–278.

Evans, J.St.B.T. (2010). Intuition and Reasoning: A dual process perspective. *Psychological Inquiry, 21*: 313–326.

Farber, B.A., Lippert, R.A., & Nevas, D.B. (1995). The therapist as attachment figure. *Psychotherapy: Theory, Research, Practice, Training, 32*(2), 204–212.

Farber, B.A., Suzuki, J.Y., & Lynch, D.A. (2019). Positive Regard and Affirmation. In Norcross, J.C. & Lambert, M.J. (Eds.). *Psychotherapy Relationships That Work: Vol.1 Evidence-Based Therapist Contributions*. (pp. 288–322). New York: Oxford University Press.

Fernyhough, C. (2017). *The voices within: the history and science of how we talk to ourselves*. London: Profile Books.

Flaskas, C. (2002). *Family therapy beyond postmodernism: Practice challenges theory*. Hove, UK/New York, USA: Brunner-Routledge.

Flaskas, C. (2005). Sticky situation, therapy mess: On impasse and the therapist's position. In Flaskas, C., Mason, B., & Perlez, A. (Eds.). *The Space Between: Experience, context, and process in the therapeutic relationship* (pp. 111–125). Londen: Karnac.

Flaskas, C. (2012). The space of reflection: thirdness and triadic relationships in family therapy. *Journal of Family Therapy*, 34, 138–156.

Framo, J. (1992). *Family-of-Origin Therapy: An intergenerational approach*. New York: Routledge.

Frankish, K. (2018). Inner Speech and Outer Thought. In Langland-Hassan, P. & Vicente, A. (Eds.). *Inner Speech: New Voices* (pp. 221–243). Oxford, UK: Oxford University Press.

Freud, S. (2012). (1912/1958). Recommendations to physicians practicing psychoanalysis. *Standard Edition*, 12, 109–120.

Friedlander, M.L., Escudero, V., & Heatherington, L. (2006). *Therapeutic Alliances in Couple and Family Therapy*. Washington, DC: American Psychological Association.

Friedlander, M.L., Escudero, V., Wilmers-van de Poll, M.J., & Heatherington, L. (2018). Meta-analysis of the alliance–outcome relation in couple and family therapy. *Psychotherapy*, 55(4), 356–371.

Friedlander, M.L., Escudero, V., Wilmers-van de Poll, M.J., & Heatherington, L. (2019). Alliance in couple and family therapy. In Norcross, J.C. & Lambert, M.J. (Eds.). *Psychotherapy Relationships that Work: Evidence-based Therapist Contributions* (3rd edition, p.117–166). New York: Oxford University Press.

Fussel, F.W. & Bonney, W.C. (1990). A comparative study of childhood experiences of psychotherapists and physicists: Implications for clinical practice. *Psychotherapy*, 27, 505–512.

Gallwey, W.T. (1974). *The Inner Game of Tennis*. New York: Random House.

Gazzaniga, M.S. (2013). Shifting Gears: Seeking new approaches for mind/brains mechanisms. *Annual Review of Psychology*, 64, 1–20.

Gelso, C.J., Kivlighan, D.M., & Markin, R.D. (2019). The Real Relationship. In Norcross, J.C. & Lambert, M.J. (Eds.). *Psychotherapy Relationships That Work: Vol.1 Evidence-Based Therapist Contributions* (pp. 351–378). New York: Oxford University Press.

Gergen, K.J. (2009). *An Invitation to Social Construction (2nd Edition)*. Los Angeles: Sage.

Glebova T. & Woolley S.R. (2016). Split Alliance in Couple and Family Therapy. In Lebow, J., Chambers, A., & Breunlin, D. (Eds.). *Encyclopedia of Couple and Family Therapy*. Cham, Switzerland: Springer.

Goffman, E. (1959). *The Presentation of Self in Everyday Life*. Garden City, New York: Doubleday, Anchor Books.

Goldberg, S.B., Rousmaniere, T., Miller, S.D., Whipple, J., Nielsen, S.L. Hoyt, W.T., & Wampold, B.E. (2016). Do Psychotherapists Improve with Time and Experience? A Longitudinal Analysis of Outcomes in a Clinical Setting. *Journal of Counseling Psychology, 1*, 1–11.

Gray, J.A. (2007). *Consciousness: Creeping up on the hard problem*. New York: Oxford University Press.

Greenberg, L.S., & Safran, J.D. (1987). *Emotion in psychotherapy: Affect, cognition, and the process of change*. New York: Guilford Press.

Greenberg, L.S. (2010). Emotion-Focused Therapy: A clinical synthesis. *Focus, 8*(1), 32–42.

Gross, J.J. & Barrett, L.F. (2011). Emotion Generation and Emotion Regulation: One or two depends on your point of view. *Emotion Review, 3*(1), 8–16.

Guerin, P.J. & Pendergast, E. (1976). Evaluation of family systems and genogram. In Guerin, P.J. (Ed.). *Family Therapy* (pp. 450–465). New York: Gardner.

Haber, R. (1990). From handicap to handy capable: Training systemic therapists in the use of self. *Family Process, 29*, 375–384.

Haber, R. & Hawley, L. (2004). Family of origin as a supervisory consultative resource. *Family Process, 43*, 373–390.

Hara, K.M., Westra, H.A., Aviram, A., Button, M.L., Constantino, M.J., & Antony, M.M. (2015). Therapist awareness of client resistance in cognitive behavioral therapy for generalized anxiety disorder. *Cognitive Behavior Therapy, 44*, 162–174.

Hardy, J. (2006). Speaking Clearly: A critical review of the self-talk literature. *Psychology of Sport and Exercise, 7*, 81–97.

Hayes, J.A. & Vinca, M. (2017). Therapist presence, absence and extraordinary presence. In Castonguay, L.G. & Hill, C.E. (Eds.). *How and Why are some therapists better than others* (pp. 85–99). Washington, DC: APA Press.

Heinonen, E. & Nissen-Lie, H.E. (2020) The professional and personal characteristics of effective psychotherapists: a systematic review. *Psychotherapy Research, 30*, 417–432.

Heyndrickx, P., De Loof, L., Knip, R., Van Herck, A., & van Kalveren, W. (2022). *Handboek Contextuele Hulpverlening: Op verhaal komen in dialoog*. Kalmthout: Pelckmans.

Herrigel, E. (1999). *Zen in the art of archery*. New York: Vintage.

Hill, C.E., Knox, S., & Pito-Coelho, K.G. (2019). Self-Disclosure and Immediacy. In Norcross, J.C. & Lambert, M.J. (Eds.). *Psychotherapy Relationships That Work - Volume 1: Evidence-Based Therapist Contributions* (pp. 379–420). New York: Oxford University Press.

Hill, C.E., Thompson, B.J., Cogar, M.C., & Denman, D.W. (1993). Beneath the surface of long-term therapy: Therapist and client report of their own and each other's covert processes. *Journal of Counseling Psychology, 40*(3), 278–287.

Hill, C.E. & Norcross, J.C. (2023). Research evidence on psychotherapist skills and methods: Foreword and afterword. *Psychotherapy Research, 33*(7), 821–840.

Hubble, M.A., Duncan, B.L., & Miller, S. (Eds.) (1999). *The Heart and Soul of Change*. Washington, DC: The American Psychological Association.

James, W. (1890, 2012). *The Principles of Psychology*. New York: Dover books.

Johns, R.G., Barkham, M., Kellett, S., & Saxon, D. (2019). A systematic review of therapist effects: A critical narrative update and refinement to Baldwin & Imel's (2013) review. *Clinical Psychology Review, 67*, 78–93.

Jurkovic, G.J. (1997). *Lost childhoods. The plight of the parentified child*. New York: Brunner-Routledge.

Kahneman, D. (2011). *Thinking fast and slow*. New York: Farrar, Straus and Giroud.

Kahneman, D. & Klein, G. (2009). Condition for intuitive expertise: A failure to disagree. *American Psychologist, 64*(6), 515–526.

Karam, E.A. & Blow, A.J. (2023). *Bringing Common Factors to Life in Couple and Family Therapy*. London: Routledge.

Keith, D. V. (1987). Intuition in family therapy: A short manual on post-modern witchcraft. *Contemporary Family Therapy, 9*, 11–22.

Keith, D.V. & Paparone, Y.Y. (2017). Training Experiential Family Therapists. In Lebow, J., Chambers, A., & Breunlin, D. (Eds.). *Encyclopedia of Couple and Family Therapy*. Cham: Springer.

Klein, G. & Hoffman, R. (2008). Macrocognition, mental models, and cognitive task analysis methodology. In Schraagen, J.M., Militello, L.G., Ormerod, T., & Lipshitz, R. (Eds.). *Naturalistic decision making and macrocognition* (pp. 57–80). Hampshire, UK: Ashgate.

Klein, G. (2004). *The Power of Intuition*. New York: Currency Books.

Klein, G. (2015). A naturalistic decision-making perspective on studying intuitive decision-making. *Journal of Applied Research in Memory and Cognition, 4*, 164–168.

Lambert, M.J. & Shimokawa, K. (2011). Collecting client feedback. *Psychotherapy: Theory, Research, Practice, Training, 48*, 72–79.

Lambert, M.J., Whipple, J.L., & Kleinstäuber, M. (2019). Collecting and Delivering Client Feedback. In Norcross, J.C. & Lambert, M.J. (Eds.). *Psychotherapy relationships that work: Vol. 1: Evidence-Based Therapist Contributions (3rd ed.)* (pp. 580–630). New York: Oxford University Press.

Langland-Hassan, P. (2021). Inner Speech. *Wiley Interdisciplinary Reviews. Cognitive Science, 12*(2), pp. e1544–n/a.

Langland-Hassan, P. & Vicente, A. (2018). Introduction. In Langland-Hassan, P. & Vicente, A. (Eds.). *Inner Speech: New Voices* (pp. 1–28). Oxford, UK: Oxford University Press.

Lappan, S., Shamoon, Z., & Blow, A. (2018). The importance of adoption of formal client feedback in therapy: A narrative review. *Journal of Family Therapy, 40*(4), 466–488.

Latinjak, A. T., Hatzigeorgiadis, A., Comoutos, N., & Hardy, J. (2019). Speaking clearly … 10 years on: The case for an integrative perspective of self-talk in sport. *Sport, Exercise, and Performance Psychology, 8*(4), 353–367.

Libet, B., Gleason, C.A., Wright, E.W., & Pearl, D.K. (1983). Time of conscious intention to act in relation to onset of cerebral activity (readiness potential): The unconscious initiation of a freely voluntary act. *Brain, 106*, 623–642.

Mahler, M., Pine, F., & Berman, A. (1975). *The psychological birth of the human infant: Symbiosis and individuation.* New York: Basic Books.

Martínez-Manrique, F. & Vicente, A. (2015). The activity view of inner speech. *Frontiers in Psychology,* 6, Article 232, 1–13.

McGoldrick, M. & Gerson, R. (1985). *Genograms in family assessment.* New York: Norton.

McRae, K. & Gross, J.J. (2020). Emotion Regulation (Introduction). *Emotion,* 20(1), 1–9.

Meehl, P.E. (1954). *Clinical versus statistical prediction: a theoretical analysis and review of the evidence.* Minneapolis: University of Minnesota Press.

Mesquita, B. (2022). *Between us: How cultures create emotions.* New York: W.W. Norton & Co.

Mikulincer, M. & Shaver, P.R. (2016). *Attachment in Adulthood: Structure, dynamics and change (2nd Edition).* New York: Guilford.

Miller, S. D., Duncan, B. L., Sparks, J. A., & Claud, D. A. (2003). The Outcome Rating Scale: A Preliminary Study of the Reliability, Validity, and Feasibility of a Brief Visual Analog Measure. *Journal of Brief Therapy,* 2(2), 91–100.

Miller, S. D., Hubble, M. A., Chow, D., & Seidel (2015). Beyond Measures and Monitoring: Realizing the potential of feedback-informed treatment. *Psychotherapy,* 52, 449–457.

Miller, S. D., Hubble, M. A., & Chow, D. (2020). *Better results: Using deliberate practice to improve therapeutic effectiveness.* Washington, DC: American Psychological Association.

Miller, W.R. & Moyers, T.B. (2021). *Effective Psychotherapists: Clinical skills that improve client outcomes.* New York: Guilford.

Minuchin, S. & Fishman, H.C. (1981). *Family Therapy Techniques.* Cambridge, Mass.: Harvard University Press.

Morgan, M.M., & Sprenkle, D.H. (2007). Toward common factors approach to supervision. *Journal of Marital and Family Therapy,* 33, 1–17.

Morin, A. (2018). The Self-Reflective Functions of Inner Speech: Thirteen Years Later. In Langland-Hassan, P. & Vicente, A. (Eds.). *Inner Speech: New Voices* (pp. 276–298). Oxford,UK: Oxford University Press.

Muran, C.J. & Eubanks, C.F. (2020). *Therapist performance under pressure: Negotiating emotions, difference, and rupture.* Washington, DC: American Psychological Association.

Newsome, J., Mitchell, L., & Awosan, C. (2018). Reframing in Couple and Family Therapy. In: Lebow, J., Chambers, A., & Breunlin, D. (Eds.). *Encyclopedia of Couple and Family Therapy.* Cham: Springer.

Nissen-Lie, H.A., Monsen, J.T., & Rønnestad, H. (2010). Therapist Predictors of early patient-rated working alliance: A multilevel approach. *Psychotherapy Research,* 20, 627–646.

Nissen-Lie, H.A., Rønnestad, M.H., Hoglend, P.A., Havik, O.E., Solbakken, O.A., Stiles, T.C., & Monsen, J.T. (2017). Love yourself as a person, doubt yourself as a therapist? *Clinical Psychology & Psychotherapy,* 24, 48–60.

Norcross, J.C. & Lambert, M.J. (2018). Psychotherapy relations that work III. *Psychotherapy,* 55, 303–315.

Norcross, J.C., & Lambert, M.J. (2019). What works in the psychotherapy relationship. In: Norcross, J.C. & Lambert, M.J. (Eds.). *Psychotherapy relationships that work: Vol. 2: Evidence-Based Therapist responsiveness (3rd ed.)* (pp. 631–646). New York: Oxford University Press.

Norcross, J. C., & Wampold, B.E. (2019). Evidence-Based Psychotherapy Responsiveness. In: Norcross, J.C. & Lambert, M.J. (Eds.). *Psychotherapy relationships that work: Vol. 2: Evidence-Based Therapist responsiveness (3rd ed.)* (pp. 1–14). New York: Oxford University Press.

Orlinsky, D.E. & Rønnestad, M.H. (2005). *How psychotherapists develop: A study of therapeutic work and professional growth.* Washington, DC: American Psychological Association.

Piaget, J. & Inhelder, B. (1966). *La Psychologie de l'Enfant.* Paris: Presses Universitaires de France.

Pinsof, W.M. (2017). The Systemic Therapy Inventory of Change—STIC: A multi-systemic and multi-dimensional system to integrate science into psychotherapeutic practice. In Tilden, T. & Wampold, B.E. (Eds.). *Routine outcome monitoring in couple and family therapy: The empirically informed therapist* (pp. 85–101). Springer International Publishing.

Plato (2014). *Theaetetus.* Oxford: Oxford University Press.

Polanyi, M. (1958). *Personal knowledge: Towards a post-critical philosophy.* London: Routledge.

Posner, M.I. & Snyder, C.R.R. (2004). Attention and cognitive control. In Bolato, D.A. & Marsh, E.J. (Eds.). *Key Readings in Cognition* (pp. 205–223). New York: Psychology Press.

Prescott, D.S. (2017). Feedback-Informed Treatment: An overview of the basics and core competencies. In Prescott, D.S., Maeschalck, C.L., & Miller, S.D. (Eds.). *Feedback-Informed Treatment in Clinical Practice* (pp. 37–52). Washington, DC: American Psychological Association.

Prescott, D.S., Maeschalck, C.L., & Miller, S.D. (Eds.). *Feedback Informed Treatment in Clinical Practice: Reaching for excellence.* Washington, DC: American Psychological Association.

Reber, A.S. (1993). *Implicit learning and tacit knowledge: An essay on the cognitive unconscious.* Oxford: Oxford University Press.

Reimers, S. (2006). Family therapy by default: Developing useful fall-back positions for therapists. *Journal of Family Therapy, 28,* 229–245.

Regas, S.J., Kostick, K.M., Bakaly, J.W., & Doonan, R.L. (2017). Including the self-of-the-therapist in clinical training. *Couple and Family Psychology: Research and Practice, 6*(1), 18–31.

Rennie, D.L. (1994). Client's deference in psychotherapy. *Journal of Counseling Psychology, 41,* 427–437.

Rhodes, R.H., Hill, C.E., Thompson, B.J., & Elliott, R. (1994). Client retrospective recall of resolved and unresolved misunderstanding events. *Journal of Counseling Psychology, 41*(4), 473–483.

Rober, P. (2005a). Family therapy as a dialogue of living persons. *Journal of Marital and Family Therapy, 31,* 385–397.

Rober, P. (2005b). The therapist's self in dialogical family therapy: Some ideas about not-knowing and the therapist's inner conversation. *Family Process, 44,* 477–495.

Rober, P. (2008). Being there, experiencing and creating space for dialogue: About working with children in family therapy. *Journal of Family Therapy, 30,* 465–477.

Rober, P. (2011). The therapist's experiencing in family therapy practice. *Journal of Family Therapy, 33,* 233–255.

Rober, P. (2012). *Gezinstherapie in Praktijk.* Leuven: Acco.

Rober, P. (2017a). Addressing the Person of the Therapist in Supervision: The Therapist's Inner Conversation Method. *Family Process, 56,* 487–500.

Rober, P. (2017b). *In Therapy Together: Family therapy as a dialogue.* London: Palgrave/Macmillan.

Rober, P. (2021). The dual process of intuitive responsivity and reflective self-supervision: About the therapist in family therapy practice. *Family Process, 60,* 1033–1047.

Rober, P., Van Tricht, K., & Sundet, R. (2021). "One step up, but not there yet": Moving towards developing a feedback-oriented family therapy. *Journal of Family Therapy, 43,* 46–53.

Rober, P. & Van Tricht, K. (2023). Using questionnaires as conversational tools to bolster the therapeutic alliance in family therapy practice. *Family Process* (accepted for publication).

Rogers, C. (1957). The Necessary and Sufficient Conditions of Therapeutic Personality Change. *Journal of Consulting Psychology, 21,* 95–103.

Rousmaniere, T. (2017). *Deliberate practice for psychotherapists: A guide to improving clinical effectiveness.* New York: Routledge.

Rousmaniere, T. (2019). *Mastering the Inner Skills of Psychotherapy: A Deliberate Practice Manual.* Gold Lantern Books.

Russon, J. & Carneiro, R. (2016). POTT principles across mental health disciplines: "just use your clinical judgment". In Aponte, H.J. & Kissil, K. (Eds.). *The Person of the Therapist Training Model: Mastering the use of self* (pp. 94–108). New York: Routledge.

Satir, V. (2013). The Therapist Story. In Baldwin, M. (Ed.). *The use of self in therapy (3rd edition)* (p.19–27). New York: Routledge.

Schachter, S. & Singer, J. (1962). Cognitive, social and psychological determinants of emotional state. *Psychological Review, 69,* 379–399.

Schön, D.A. (1983). *The Reflective Practitioner: How professionals think in action.* New York: Basic Books.

Schöttke, H., Flückiger, C., Goldberg, S.B., Eversman, J., & Lange, J. (2017). Predicting psychotherapy outcome based on therapist interpersonal skills: A five-year longitudinal study of a therapist assessment protocol. *Psychotherapy Research, 27,* 642–652.

Scott, L. & Wendt, D. (2018). Self of the therapist training in couple and family therapy. In Lebow, J.L., Chambers, A., & Breunlin, D.C. (Eds.). *Encyclopedia of Couple and Family Therapy.* New York: Springer International Publishing.

Shimokawa, K., Lambert, M. J., & Smart, D. W. (2010). Enhancing treatment outcome of patients at risk of treatment failure: meta-analytic and mega-analytic review of a psychotherapy quality assurance system. *Journal of Consulting and Clinical Psychology*, 78(3), 298–311.

Shotter, J. (2016). *Speaking, Actually: Towards a new fluid common-sense understanding of relational becomings.* Farnhill, UK: Everything is Connected Press.

Simon, G. (2006). The heart of the matter: A proposal for placing the self of the therapist at the center of family therapy research and training. *Family Process*, 45, 331–344.

Soloski, K.L., Turns, B., Schleiden, C., & Macey, P. (2016). Parentified Child in Family Systems. In Lebow, J., Chambers, A., & Breunlin, D. (Eds). *Encyclopedia of Couple and Family Therapy.* Cham: Springer.

Soma, C.S., Baucom, B.R.W., Xiao, B., Butner, J.E., Hilpert, P., Narayanan, S., Atkins, D.C., & Imel, Z.E. (2020) Coregulation of therapist and client emotion during psychotherapy, *Psychotherapy Research*, 30(5), 591–603.

Stanovic, K.E. & West, R.F. (2000). Individual differences in reasoning: Implications for the rationality debate? *Behavioral and Brain Science*, 23, 645–665.

Stern, D.N. (1985). *The Interpersonal World of The Infant: A view from psychoanalysis and developmental psychology.* New York: Basic Books.

Stern, D.N. (2004). *The Present Moment in Psychotherapy and Everyday Life.* New York: Norton.

Stock, B. (2018). *Augustine's Inner Dialogue: The Philosophical soliloquy in Late Antiquity.* Cambridge, UK: Cambridge University Press.

Stratton, P., Bland, J., James, E., & Lask, J. (2010). Developing an indicator of family function and a practicable outcome measure for systemic and couple therapy: The SCORE. *Journal of Family Therapy*, 32, 232–258.

Sun, R. (2015). Interpreting psychological notions: A dual process computational theory. *Journal of Applied Research in Memory and Cognition*, 4, 191–196.

Sundet, R. (2011). Collaboration: family and therapist perspectives of helpful therapy. *Journal of Marital and Family Therapy*, 37(2), 236–249.

Sundet, R. (2014). Patient focused research supported practices in an intensive family therapy unit. *Journal of Family Therapy*, 36, 195–216.

Sundet, R. (2017). Feedback as a means to enhance client-therapist interaction in therapy. In Tilden, T. & Wampold, B. (Eds.). *Routing Outcome Monitoring in Couple and Family Therapy* (pp. 121–142). Cham, Switzerland: Springer.

Tilden, T. & Wampold, B. (2017) (Eds.). *Routing Outcome Monitoring in Couple and Family Therapy.* Cham, Switzerland: Springer.

Timm, T.M. & Blow, A.J. (1999). Self-of-the-therapist work: A balance between removing restraints and identifying resources. *Contemporary Family Therapy*, 21, 331–350.

Tod, D., Hardy, J., & Oliver, E.J. (2011). Effects of self-talk: A systematic review. *Journal of Sports and Exercise Psychology*, 33, 666–687.

Tryon, G.S., Birch, S.E., & Verkuilen, J. (2019). Goal Consensus and Collaboration. In Norcross, J.C. & Lambert, M.J. (Eds.). *Psychotherapy*

*Relationships That Work: Vol.1 Evidence-Based Therapist Contributions* (pp. 167–204). New York: Oxford University Press.

van Oenen, F., Schipper, S., Van, R, Schoevers, R. Visch, I., Peen, J., & Dekker, J. (2016). Feedback-informed treatment in emergency psychiatry: a randomized controlled trial. *BMC Psychiatry*, 16, 110–110.

Van Raalte, J.L., Vincent, A., & Brewer, B.W. (2016). Self talk: Review and sport specific model. *Psychology of Sport and Exercise*, 22, 139–148.

Varela, F.J., Rosch, E., & Thompson, E. (1992). *The Embodied Mind: Cognitive Science and Human Experience*. Cambridge, MA: MIT Press.

Vygotsky, L.S. (1962). *Thought and Language*. Cambridge, Mass.: The M.I.T Press.

Walfish, S., McAlister, B., O'Donnell, P., & Lambert, M.J. (2012). An investigation of self-assessment bias in mental health providers. *Psychological Reports*, 110, 639–644.

Wampold, B.E. & Imel, Z.E. (2015). *The Great Psychotherapy Debate: The evidence for what makes psychotherapy work*. New York: Routledge.

Wampold, B.E. (2015). How important are the common factors in psychotherapy? An update. *World Psychiatry*, 14, 270–277.

Wampold, B.E. (2017). What should we practice: A contextual model for how psychotherapy works. In Rousmaniere, T., Goodyear, R.K., Miller, S.D., & Wampold, B.E. (Eds.). *The Cycle of Excellence: using deliberate practice to improve supervision and training* (pp. 49–65). Hoboken, NJ: Willey Blackwell.

Wampold, B.E., Baldwin, S.A., Holtforth, M.G., & Imel, Z.E. (2017). What characterizes effective therapists? In Castonguay, L.G. & Hill, C.E. (Eds). *How and why are some therapists better than others? Understanding therapist effects* (pp. 37–53). Washington, DC: American Psychological Association.

Wampold, B.E. & Owens, J. (2021). Therapist effects: History, methods, magnitude and characteristics of effective therapists. In Barkham, M., Lutz, W., & Castonguay, L.G. (Eds.). *Bergin and Garfield's Handbook of Psychotherapy and Behavior Change* (pp. 297–326). Hoboken, NJ: Wiley.

Watson, J.C. & Wiseman, H. (Eds.) (2021). *The Responsive Psychotherapist: Attuning to clients in the moment*. Washington, DC: American Psychological Association.

Webb, C.A., DuRubeis, R.J., & Barber, J.P. (2010). Therapist adherence/competence and treatment outcome: A meta-analytic review. *Journal of Consulting and Clinical Psychology*, 78(2), 299–310.

Westen, D. & Weinberger, J. (2005). In praise of clinical judgment: Meehl's forgotten legacy. *Journal of Clinical Psychology*, 61(10), 1257–1276.

Westra, H.A., Aviram, A., Connors, L., Kertes, A., & Ahmed, M. (2012). Therapist emotional reactions and client resistance in cognitive behavioral therapy. *Psychotherapy*, 49, 163–172.

Whitaker, C. A., Warkentin, J., & Johnson, N. (1950). The psychotherapeutic impasse. *American Journal of Orthopsychiatry*, 20(3), 641–647.

Whitaker, C. & Keith, D.V. (1980). Symbolic-Experiential Family Therapy. In Gurman, A. & Kniskern, P. (Eds.). *Handbook of Family Therapy* (p. 187–225). New York: Bruner/Mazel.

White, M. (2007). *Maps of Narrative Practice*. New York: Norton.

White, M. (2000). Re-engaging with history: The absent but implicit. In White, M. (Ed.). *Reflections on narrative practice* (pp. 35–58). Adelaide, South Australia: Dulwich Centre Publications.

Wiley, N. (2016). *Inner Speech and the Dialogical Self*. Philadelphia: Temple University Press.

Wilkinson, S. & Fernyhough, C. (2018). When Inner Speech Misleads. In Langland-Hassan, P. & Vicente, A. (Eds.). *Inner Speech: New Voices* (pp. 244–260). Oxford, UK: Oxford University Press.

Wilson, J. (2007). *The Performance of Practice: Enhancing the Repertoire of the Family Therapist*. London: Karnac Books.

Wolf, W.A., Goldfried, M.R., & Muran, J.C. (2017). Therapist negative reactions: How to transform toxic experiences. In Castonguay, L.G. & Hill, C.E. (Eds.). *How and why are some therapists better than others? Understanding therapist effects* (pp. 175–192). Washington, DC: American Psychological Association.

Yalom, I. (1980). *Existential Psychotherapy*. New York: Basic Books.

Zerubavel, N., & Wright, M.O.D. (2012). The dilemma of the wounded healer. *Psychotherapy, 49*(4), 482–491.

# Attachment 1: The Worries Questionnaire

## (WQ - Rober & Van Tricht, 2015)

Name: .........................................

Date: .........................................

Who in your family is the most worried at the moment?
- □ me
- □ someone else....................................................................

How worried is that (most worried) person at this moment on a scale from 0 to 10 (when "0" means "not worried at all" and "10" means "extremely worried")?

| 0 | 1 | 2 | 3 | 4 | 5 | 6 | 7 | 8 | 9 | 10 |
|---|---|---|---|---|---|---|---|---|---|----|

Can you describe in a few sentences what the most worried person is concerned about?

Can you describe in a few sentences why the most worried person thinks therapy can be useful or not useful at this moment?

```



```

If you are not the most worried family member, how worried are you at this moment on a scale from 0 to 10 (when "0" means "not worried at all" and "10" means "extremely worried")?

| 0 | 1 | 2 | 3 | 4 | 5 | 6 | 7 | 8 | 9 | 10 |
|---|---|---|---|---|---|---|---|---|---|----|

If you are not the most worried family member, can you describe in a few sentences what you are concerned about?

```



```

If you are not the most worried family member, can you describe in a few sentences why you think therapy can be useful at this moment; or why you think it might not be usefull?

```



```

(WQ - p.2/2)

# Attachment 2: The Dialogical Feedback Questionnaire
## (DFQ - Rober & Van Tricht, 2015)

Name: ......................................

Date: ...........................................

1. Were you able to talk about what you wanted in the session?

| 0 | 1 | 2 | 3 | 4 | 5 | 6 | 7 | 8 | 9 | 10 |
|---|---|---|---|---|---|---|---|---|---|----|

*Not at all*                                                      *Totally*

A word of explanation:

2. Did you feel understood by the therapist(s) during the session?

| 0 | 1 | 2 | 3 | 4 | 5 | 6 | 7 | 8 | 9 | 10 |
|---|---|---|---|---|---|---|---|---|---|----|

*Not at all*                                                      *Totally*

| In this area I didn't feel understood: | In this area I felt understood: |
|---|---|
|  |  |

(DFQ p.1/2)

3. Did you feel understood by your partner / the other family members during the session?

| 0 | 1 | 2 | 3 | 4 | 5 | 6 | 7 | 8 | 9 | 10 |
|---|---|---|---|---|---|---|---|---|---|----|

*Not at all*                                                                 *Totally*

| In this area I didn't feel understood: | In this area I felt understood: |
|---|---|
| | |

4. What *surprised* you most during the session?

| |
|---|
| |

5. What *moved* you most during the session?

| |
|---|
| |

(DFQ p.2/2)

# Attachment 3: Self-supervision Questionnaire (for family therapy) (SSQ-FT, Rober & Van Tricht, 2020)

Name therapist: .............................

Date: .............................

Name family: .............................

**1. The conversation went smooth. The family members talked freely with each other (and with me) about their hesitations and their worries.**

| 0 | 1 | 2 | 3 | 4 | 5 | 6 | 7 | 8 | 9 | 10 |
|---|---|---|---|---|---|---|---|---|---|----|

Not at all                                                              Totally

| A word of explanation: |
|---|
|  |

**2. I felt attuned to the family and I connected well with each of the family members.**

| 0 | 1 | 2 | 3 | 4 | 5 | 6 | 7 | 8 | 9 | 10 |
|---|---|---|---|---|---|---|---|---|---|----|

Not at all                                                              Totally

| I was not attuned to these family members: | I was well attuned to these family members: |
|---|---|
|  |  |

(SSQ, 1/2)

**3. I felt comfortable as a therapist. I did not feel any pressure and I had no specific worries.**

| 0 | 1 | 2 | 3 | 4 | 5 | 6 | 7 | 8 | 9 | 10 |

Not at all                                                                Totally

| I felt pressure and I was worried about... | I felt comfortable and I experienced that I could be of help for this family by... |
|---|---|
|  |  |

**4. This *surprised* me most during the session.**

|  |
|---|
|  |

**5. This *moved* me most during the session.**

|  |
|---|
|  |

(SSQ, 2/2)

# Index

Note: Locators in *italic* indicate figures and in ***bold italic*** boxes.

For Product Safety Concerns and Information please contact our EU
representative GPSR@taylorandfrancis.com
Taylor & Francis Verlag GmbH, Kaufingerstraße 24, 80331 München, Germany